A Break in the Storm

Coping with Major Depression

By Ron Fritz

A Break in the Storm
Coping with Major Depression
By Ron Fritz, MS

Copyright © 2017 by Ron Fritz

Published by RAE Publishing
Printed by CreateSpace, An Amazon.com Company

Send Correspondance to:
Ron Fritz
P.O. Box 72254
Phoenix, AZ 85050

ISBN: 978-0692049617
Cover photography provided by Donna Fritz

Printed in the United States

Dedication

This book is dedicated to the many depressives who silently suffer from the scorn of the Beast. May you find comfort and solace in these pages.

This Page left Intentionally Blank

Table of Contents

Forward

I have been a depressive since 1971; I was 11 years old. I didn't know at the time I had depression, I just knew I felt different than the rest of the kids my age. I just assumed I was strange.

I was first diagnosed with depression by a NAVY doctor when I was 22. At last this thing had a name. I also met my first depressive (other than myself) when I was 22. It was liberating, I was no longer alone. There were other strange people in the world too.

I treated my depression with alcohol and it worked for a while. Eventually it stopped working. I quit drinking alcohol in 1987; I was 27 years old. I am thankful to the people at Baker House, the treatment center I went to; they saved my life. I only wish they had known more about depression, because once I became sober my depression returned; I just didn't have any coping skills for my depression. That was a very difficult time in my life.

I dove into studying about Depression, I had to learn my enemy. I've always excelled at school and I studied depression until I became an expert. I've been studying the Beast now for 30 years; I'm still learning new things about him.

Over the years I have worked with hundreds (possibly thousands) of depressives. I have helped well over a hundred suicidal individuals, and dozens of families of suicide victims. I can relate to them, and I don't judge them.

In 1996 I met my wife. She is the love of my life. When we first met I told her I suffered from depression and she just smiled. She later admitted to me that she had no idea what it really meant to have

9

depression; she was a normie. As my episodes came and went, she learned how bad it could get, and as she learned, she became adept at helping me during my low points. My wife is an Angel. She must be, because she has helped me fight the Beast.

My first real therapist, Heather, suggested I write this book. She thought it would be therapeutic. She was right, it has been. I owe Heather my gratitude for helping me through a rough time. My wife Donna is the biggest hero in this story, because she stood by me as I wrote, she proofread over and over, and she has encouraged me to finish this book. This book would not exist were it not for her confidence in me and her unfailing support.

I hope this book helps you get to tomorrow.

Ron

Chapter 1
Living in the Fog
What Does Depression Feel Like?

Sitting on the beach with the sun overhead, I see a fog forming over the ocean. Even though the fog is in the distance, it appears sadly ominous and goose bumps rise on my arms. Looking around, no one else seems to notice the approaching fog and it occurs to me they might not be able to see it.

As the fog rolls in closer, it swallows up every boat in its path. I watch the people furthest from me gradually become hazy and difficult to see, until they finally become obscured altogether. It feels as if the world is shrinking. There is no clear point where I'm aware the fog has enveloped me. Every time this happens I tell myself I will watch for the point when the fog takes me, and each time I become so focused on the boats disappearing that before I realize what's happening, the light is gone.

At first the fog is wispy, its tentacles snatching at my limbs as it strives to control me. I do my best to ignore the approaching fog and sense it is laughing at me for denying it. I want to believe if I just pretend the fog doesn't exist that perhaps this time it won't come. In my heart, I know better. The fog continues to thicken and as it does, the people around me move further away.

They don't seem to know what's happening and I realize I'm the one who is retreating. The fog begins to assume a presence,

11

as if it is standing between me and the rest of the world. I feel it surrounding me and taking control. I want to push it away, and yet I discover I haven't the strength.

The fog has weight. The thicker the fog becomes, the heavier the weight that it piles on my shoulders. It's no coincidence that thick fog is often referred to as heavy fog; it presses down on my shoulders and becomes a burden I can actually feel. The fog restrains me. The fog holds me down and makes every movement an effort of sheer will. The fog is exhausting, and it saps my strength. Most of all, the fog is relentless.

The fog grows thicker and I know the darkness is inevitable. It has replaced everything and wherever I turn, it is there. Escape is futile because there is no place to run. I can no longer see anyone around me, and hear only the sound of faint voices. The fog has swallowed me and I'm completely alone. No one knows I'm missing. The worst kind of lost is when you know that no help is coming. No one is looking for you.

There is no fighting the fog. No way out. My only hope is that the fog will pass, just as it has before. The weight seems unbearable and any movement requires tremendous effort. All I can do is curl up in the fetal position and wait for the fog to leave.

My First Glimpse of Depression

The first time I remember feeling the depression, I was 11 years old. Most people find it difficult to believe that an 11-year boy old can be depressed. "What does an 11-year old have to be depressed about?" they ask. I tell them it's not "about something," the depression simply is. I've learned that people who don't have depression have a hard time understanding this.

When I was 11, my grandmother killed herself. She decided she did not want to do life anymore and she took a bottle full of pills. I didn't feel sad. I knew I'd miss her; I was very close to my grandmother. However, there was no reason for me to be sad because everyone said my grandmother wasn't in any more pain; that she had gone to a better place. When I was 11 years old I learned that death was a better place than living.

My parents took me to see my grandmother in the "viewing room." She looked very peaceful and my mother told me that grandma was resting. It's funny; people refer to dying as "resting" and being buried as "going to the final resting place" and yet they get all bent out of shape when someone commits suicide so he or she can go there. I hoped my grandmother was happier. I can remember feeling very disconnected that day, as if I was in a dream. It was a feeling I would become very familiar with the rest of my life.

Living on an Island

To my best recollection, that was the day I started to isolate myself from the world. I became an island, and oddly enough, no one seemed to notice. Looking back, I realize that was the day the fog started to roll in. It didn't happen all at once; it slowly crept in over several years. Because it was the first time, I had no idea what was happening. All I knew was that the way I looked at the world seemed to be changing.

Being alone was more comfortable than being with people. I'm not sure if I pushed others away or if they just avoided me because I was different; I just never felt like I belonged. It seemed as if everyone was in on a secret, and I was the only one who didn't know what the secret was. I could see others having fun and I longed to have fun too, however, I didn't seem to get the same enjoyment from activities that others did. It felt as if there was a dark black cloud overshadowing me, chasing away any potential joy I might hope to experience.

I started crying during those years. Most people cry because they feel sad or are in pain. I would start crying when I became angry, when I felt powerless, when I was embarrassed, or when I felt threatened. Occasionally, I would cry for no reason at all. I could be watching a movie or in the middle of a conversation and the tears would start to fall. Sometimes I didn't even realize I was crying until someone pointed it out.

I cried a lot and I hated myself for it; men aren't supposed to cry. We're taught from a young age that crying is a weakness and I felt self-loathing every time I did it. It was beyond my control and that bothered me more than anything. Excusing myself to go to the restroom so I could hide my tears became a common occurrence. I rehearsed many excuses: something in my eye, allergies, the wind,

14

none of them were true. Quickness to cry was something that would haunt me my whole life, and I eventually learned that the higher my depression was, the easier it became for me to break down in tears.

The local movie theater became my refuge. I spent hour after hour watching movies I cared nothing about and eating popcorn I didn't want. Sometimes I would show up for the first matinee and stay until the theater closed, watching the same movie over and over. What I liked most about the theater was that you could be in a room full of people and still be entirely alone. You didn't have to talk to anyone and no one knew you were there. It felt safe.

In Search of Safety

Safety is a big issue for someone with depression. Darkness is safe. Small spaces feel safe. Being alone feels safe. When someone is experiencing depression, the last thing he or she wants, is to be around a lot of people. Large parties with lots of people mingling, and everyone talking at once, can lead someone with depression into a full-blown panic attack.

My favorite safe place is an empty house where I can turn off all the lights, close the curtains, and hide curled up in a closet with the door closed and a blanket pulled over me. To someone without depression, this probably seems a little strange; to someone with depression, it will seem safe. Safety means you can't be seen; you can't be found.

People with depression don't fear the same things that normal people fear. Most people fear death; sometimes individuals suffering from depression pray for it. People with Major Depression fear living because life is exhausting when you're always waiting for the next fog to roll in.

Often depressives are obsessed with death. Many people with Major Depression obsess about death and suicide; some read about it, a few even study it. A fascination with death only reinforces the depressive's feeling about being different. Personally, I have always found cemeteries comforting because they are full of people who have found peace. I have known many depressives who shared my feelings regarding graveyards.

Our biggest fear is that someone will know our thoughts. We realize our thoughts are not normal and we live in constant fear that someone will find us out. Depression is so misunderstood that usually depressive individuals have no one they can confide in, no one with whom they can share their thoughts. Depression is a lonely secret.

The Storm Hits with Full Fury

By age 17 my depression had enveloped me completely. It ruled my life and obscured everything around me. I began to feel as if I was just marking time, waiting for the next day to come, with no hope of tomorrow becoming any better than today. I lost interest in most activities except for drama, movies, and books. These diversions allowed me to become someone else for a short time and escape my own dreary and worthless existence.

I also began drinking more. I discovered several years earlier that drinking alcohol seemed to make my feelings of worthlessness go away, albeit only for a short time. As my depression increased, so did my drinking; alcohol was my attempt to chase back the fog. I'll talk more about the relationship between drinking alcohol and depression in Chapter 7; for now, let's just say that the relief alcohol provides from depression is temporary, and eventually disappears altogether.

When I turned 17, my depression moved to a whole new level; I began thinking about suicide. At first they were just fleeting thoughts like, "What if I swerved across the lane and hit that semitruck coming toward me head-on?" Suicidal thoughts can seduce you. When every day is filled with emotional pain, the thought of not having to go through it again tomorrow can have a very calming effect.

Eventually the seduction was complete, and I made the decision to kill myself. I had been experiencing some problems at school, and although by itself, this wasn't enough to cause me to decide to kill myself, it did cement the belief I had developed that life was not worth the pain. Once I made the decision to commit suicide, the where, when, and how were just details.

I lived in a small town in the mountains, and I decided the easiest way to kill myself would be to drive my truck off one of the numerous nearby cliffs. That way I reasoned, my parents could just believe I had fallen asleep at the wheel, and would be spared any guilt they might try to assume. I decided on Saturday night, and having made the decision, found myself feeling surprisingly more upbeat than I had been in a long time. As the day approached, I found myself frequently telling my family I loved them; although they never knew it, I was telling them goodbye.

When Saturday night arrived, I bought a six-pack of beer and headed toward the cliffs. I drove by my chosen spot and continued for another 30 minutes. My plan was to drink the beer for courage, and to lend credibility to my having fallen asleep at the wheel, and then start back and have my "accident" on the return trip. As I sat drinking beer in the dark, I contemplated how life worked for some people, but I wasn't one of them. When I was sufficiently buzzed, I headed back toward the cliff.

The location I chose was a curve in the highway with a dirt pullout on the side, and no railing between the pullout and a drop of several hundred feet. It was the kind of location that is an accident waiting to happen. As I drove along the dark highway toward my destination, I thought about my life so far. There were many things I wanted to do that I still hadn't accomplished. I was 17 and I had never even kissed a girl. I mentally began ticking off things in my 'bucket list' that I wished I had done.

As the curve came into view I began accelerating. I would fly off that cliff like a rocket being launched into space. I had no doubt that the height would be more than sufficient to kill me, and I undid my seat belt for added insurance. As I sped closer toward the cliff, my mind was immediately flooded with the list I had compiled of the things I still wanted to do. "Why was I in such a hurry?" In my semi-drunken state, I convinced myself that I had a right to kiss a girl before I died.

As my pickup truck left the pavement and hit the dirt pullout, I slammed on the brakes. The brakes locked up and the truck went into a skid. The dirt pullout provided poor traction for the brakes, and the truck moved quickly toward the edge of the cliff. I locked my arms and braced myself. Just as I thought this was it, my truck slid to a stop about 10 feet from the cliff's edge. As I sat in my truck with my headlights staring ahead into space, I felt shame for having failed.

My first thought was that I couldn't do anything right. I consoled myself with the notion that this didn't mean I wouldn't kill myself, just that I wouldn't do it that night. People who have never been suicidal usually don't grasp the idea that when you've lost control of everything else in your life, the time and manner you check out is the one thing you have left that you can control. I simply told myself that I would choose a different time and place to kill myself.

As I drove home in the dark, I silently promised myself I would talk to no one about what had happened. I knew in my heart that nobody would understand and that if I admitted to anyone what I tried to do, they would think I was crazy; they would also try to talk me out of doing it again. The fog is very cunning. When you have depression, the thing you most need is to talk to someone, and the fog convinces you that is the worst thing you can do. I believed if others knew my thoughts they would want to lock me up. I vowed to keep my depression a secret.

The Need for Secrecy

Secrecy is another big issue for someone with depression. The stigma surrounding depression and suicide is so great that many depressive individuals live in fear that someone will find out their secret. When someone commits suicide, there is usually a great deal of, "How could he do this to his family?" or, "She was selfish for taking her own life." Depressive individuals come to believe their thoughts are wrong and that they will be condemned, or looked down upon by anyone who learns the truth.

People with depression become very good at hiding it. They must because they believe the rest of the world expects it. When you tell most people that you're having a depressive episode, they react by telling you they'll help "cheer you up." I want to scream every time I hear those words. When so few people understand what depression is, can anyone blame us for not wanting to disclose how we are feeling?

I learned to put a mask on my depression very early, and I could turn it on and off at will. Most of the time I left the mask on because it was too hard to explain if someone saw me without it. Normal people expect others to be happy, because it reinforces their own good feelings. I learned to smile and give others the response they were looking for; it was less work then explaining why I was always down. I usually only allowed the mask to come off when I was alone; when I was safe.

Depression Returns Like an Unwelcome Guest

After my encounter with the cliff, things got better ... for a while. The fog lifted. It became easy to forget just how dark my life had been. The depression stayed away for about 4 to 5 years and then one day ... the fog peeked over the horizon. Before that day, I felt like I was riding on top of the world. Seeing my vulnerability, the depression came on like a storm gale, and brought me crashing back down to the ground.

My depression became much deeper than I experienced during my previous episode. It swallowed me up and I retreated from everyone that even remotely cared about me. I came to believe that if I stepped off the planet, no one would notice I was gone. That was exactly what I longed to do. I began to fantasize about a deserted island where I was completely alone. No problems, no stress, just blissful solitude. I also began to fantasize about dying.

By age 27 my depression had become intolerable. My drinking increased as I became a full-fledged alcoholic. Eventually the alcohol stopped providing relief from my depression. The fog just laughed at me. I received my 4th DUI and experienced hopelessness like I had never felt before. I became convinced that this was all my life would ever amount to, a pitiful and despondent drunk.

I went home after being charged at the police station with a DUI, and I proceeded to fill the bathtub full of water. I plugged in my hair dryer and sat on the edge of the bathtub to try to remember how to pray. As I thought about how everything would be better in a few minutes, I passed out from the excessive alcohol in my system; or perhaps God knocked me out.

I woke up in the morning on the edge of the bathtub with a hairdryer in my hand; I realized this was not normal. I bleakly called my mother and asked her to meet me for coffee. When we met at the restaurant, I didn't tell her about my near electrocution, I didn't dare. Instead I told her my drinking was out of control and I needed help. She helped me check into a rehab center that day and I have not taken a drink since.

The depression got better again ... for a while. I wasn't naïve enough this time to think the fog would stay away forever. I began learning about my depression. I learned what I had was a disorder, that there was a reason for it. I learned that I wasn't alone. I learned there were things I could do to fight my depression. I was in control again for about four years, and then the fog returned.

I also learned what it looks like when the depression is coming back. I begin to care less and less about things that have previously been important to me. I begin avoiding people who are close to me;

I don't want them to see what is happening. I start avoiding outdoor activities and I find solace in the darkness.

When the next storm hit, it came with a fury. I braced myself and prayed to God to let me die in my sleep. When the storm finally peaked, I locked myself in my house, living and sleeping in a closet, only coming out in the middle of the night to use the bathroom and eat. The closet was safe. In the closet I reacquainted myself with my depression. When I finally left the closet after seven days, the fog was retreating.

I've had four more depressive episodes since then ... so far. I have learned that depression comes and goes in cycles. When my depression goes away, life is good. When my depression hits, I become lost. I don't like planning for the distant future; I focus on planning for tomorrow. I've learned that the things I most do not want to do, like getting out in the sun, talking to people, and making myself start new projects, are the things I most need to do. I've learned that if I can hang on, the fog will pass.

This Page left Intentionally Blank

Chapter 2
Depression Is Such
a Wimpy Word
Battling the Misunderstanding of Others

Everyone experiences normal depression at some time in his or her life. What is normal depression? Normal depression is usually caused by a life-changing event such as the death of a loved one, or the loss of a job. Typically, something triggers the depression and it can last anywhere from a few days to six months, e.g. in some cases of grieving.

Normal depression will usually leave people feeling like they have no energy, no desire to participate in activities they normally enjoy, and in general, feeling depressed. It's common for people with normal depression to want to sleep more, eat less, and spend less time with others. Normal depression generally goes away on its own in a relatively short time without the need for medication or treatment.

Everyone understands normal depression because it's a feeling most people have felt. When someone is experiencing normal depression, that person is often described as blue, cheerless, down, dreary, gloomy, heavy-hearted, in the dumps, low, melancholy, sad, sorrowful, or just plain unhappy. Using any of these words to describe someone who suffers from Major Depression is akin to describing someone with a migraine as having a headache.

25

The fact that most people have experienced normal depression makes it difficult for them to understand Major Depression. Because they have experienced normal depression and recovered from it on their own, they assume someone with Major Depression is going through something similar and should also be able to "get over it." Many of these people believe that medication is unnecessary, and is simply used as a crutch. They couldn't be more wrong.

Major Depression vs. Normal Depression

Major Depression is nothing like normal depression. Someone with Major Depression may feel completely worthless, hopeless, and empty. They may feel lost and alone. They may not receive any enjoyment from life's many pleasures. They may believe life is no longer worth living. Sometimes they even feel suicidal. Depression is such a wimpy word for what we go through.

It's difficult for someone who doesn't have Major Depression to empathize with the feelings and emotions a depressive has. That doesn't stop them from trying (bless their little hearts). I've lost count of the number of times I told someone I suffered from depression only to hear in response, "I know what that feels like, I got really depressed when my mother (brother, friend, favorite cat) died." Although I sympathize with their loss, it's not the same thing.

When someone with Major Depression dares to confide his or her depression in others, the individual typically hears a list of suggestions the other person recommends for depression. These suggestions can range from the ridiculous, "Think happy thoughts," or "Get a good night sleep and you'll feel better tomorrow," to the completely absurd, "Tell yourself you refuse to be depressed" or "Just snap out of it." Someone with Major Depression in the middle of a depressive episode can no more "snap out of it" than someone with cancer can spontaneously heal him or herself.

People with Major Depression learn to keep their depression to themselves because of the lack of compassion and understanding normal people have toward them. "Normal people" is how depressives refer to individuals who don't suffer from Major Depression. Normal people are happy most of the time. Normal people like to have happy people around them.

Individuals with Major Depression are sometimes accused of "killing the mood" or "bringing everyone down." Most depressives learn to wear a mask to hide their depression so normal people won't berate them, or worse, try to cheer them up. The problem with hiding behind a mask is that sometimes others don't realize how serious the depressive's condition is until it's too late.

Depression is a Chronic Mental Illness

Major Depression is an illness. It is as much an illness as cancer, hepatitis, HIV, or Heart Disease. Like these other illnesses, Major Depression can also kill you. A primary difference between Major Depression and these other illnesses is that individuals with Major Depression are often reluctant to seek help or even admit to others the nature of their illness. Just as HIV compromises an individual's immune system over time, depression episodes make it increasingly difficult for the depressive to make decisions, handle stress, and in general, deal with life.

The Center for Disease Control and Prevention (CDC) reports more than 42,000 people in the United States die from suicide every year.[1] The CDC also reports suicide is the second leading cause of death in the age groups 15-24 and 25-34.[2] For someone with Major Depression, suicide is sometimes viewed as the only way to end the individual's suffering.

Even if someone isn't suicidal, depression takes a toll on health and wellness. Individuals with Major Depression historically get less exercise, have poor eating habits, and generally don't get enough sleep. Symptoms of Major Depression include lack of energy, and loss of interest in pleasurable activities.[3] Major Depression can also lead to additional health problems, such as increased risk of heart attack or cardiovascular disease.[4] Finally, Major Depression can lead to alcoholism or drug addiction.

Major Depression is a chronic illness. When an illness is Chronic, it means the condition persists for a long time. Major Depression is also called Clinical Depression or Major Depressive Disorder (MDD). People afflicted with MDD may experience recurrences throughout the rest of their lives. Depressive episodes can last for months, sometimes even years. A primary goal in the treatment of MDD is minimizing the severity and length of depression relapses.

One of the biggest obstacles to treating Major Depression is the reluctance of those who suffer from MDD, confiding in someone about their problem. The very nature of the illness makes it difficult for those afflicted, from seeking help. Feelings of worthlessness, an inability to make good decisions, and an overwhelming desire to be alone, all prove to be major barriers to the depressive individual consulting a professional.

Major Depression is a mental illness. The phrase "mental illness" conjures up any number of horrific images for a large portion of the population. Images such as padded rooms and patients wearing straight-jackets. The stigma attached to having a "mental illness" is so powerful that individuals with MDD are often encouraged by family members, friends, and employers to keep quiet about their condition. Many depressives come to believe that they have two choices, to keep their depression a secret, or tell others and become an outcast.

The Stigma Surrounding Depression

Many people suffering from Major Depression avoid seeking help because of the enormous stigma associated with the illness. Depressives are frequently told by people who know nothing about the disorder, that overcoming depression simply requires a strong will. Unfortunately, after hearing this, the individual comes to think of his or her depression as a weakness. These individuals tend to feel inferior to those around them, and tell themselves they should be able to handle their depression on their own.

Fear of being judged, discriminated against, or simply avoided altogether convinces many depressives to hide their depression from the rest of the world. Equally as devastating to the person who has Major Depression, is the common belief among normal people that depression is simply imagined, or even worse, is nothing more than an attempt to gain attention.

No one would ever accuse someone with Leukemia of getting cancer to gain attention, yet many people don't think twice about telling a someone that their depression is imagined. Major Depression is no more an attempt to gain attention than is having Leukemia.

Sadly, individuals with Major Depression are confronted with negative stereotypes so often, they begin to convince themselves the stereotypes are true. Print and visual media often associate depression with failure and weakness. Men who cry on television are portrayed as effeminate and fragile. News reporters discuss suicides flippantly, with little to no compassion for the individual who killed him or herself, and what they may have gone through. The prevalent message individuals with Major Depression receive is, "Don't talk about your depression or people will condemn you for it." For many depressives, these become words to live by.

From a Depressive's Viewpoint

If someone were to walk in my shoes for even a single month, that person would abandon any thought that depression equates to weakness. It sometimes feels as if superhuman strength is required to endure the trials my depression places on me. Living with depression requires courage ... courage to face the Beast even when you know it intends to devour you.

When normal people hear that someone has suicidal thoughts, they often react with, "How could he (or she) even think that?" They never seem to realize the point is ... he (or she) didn't act on those thoughts. To someone who is suicidal, killing themselves seems like a solution to all their problems. To contemplate suicide and not act requires tremendous courage. The stigma that surrounds suicide is so great that it often prevents a suicidal individual from confiding in anyone. Most suicidal individuals keep their thoughts secret from those around them.

I have lost count of the nights I fell asleep praying that I would not wake up the next morning; it must number in the thousands. When I wake up the next morning and realize, once again, my prayers were not answered, I muster every ounce of strength I have and prepare myself for another day. Depression, and the stigma that goes with it, prevent individuals with MDD from calling out for help. Depression is a huge burden to carry. My depression lies to me. My depression tells me I'm worthless. My depression tells me no one wants me around. To walk through the fog alone requires tremendous courage; you never know what's up ahead.

I am always amused when people tell me that I seem too happy to suffer from depression. Their comment tells me that I have learned to wear my mask well. The stigma associated with depression leads individuals with MDD to hide their depression from everyone around them. Depressives learn to put their cheerful mask on and off at will; some individuals with MDD never take the mask off. Often family members and coworkers are completely unaware of their loved one or coworker's depression. Most people who suffer from Major Depression are very good actors.

History of Treating Depression

Depression has been around since humans first learned to hide in caves to escape the rain. Many famous figures in history can be identified who most likely suffered from depression; figures such as Virginia Woolf, Ernest Hemingway, Abraham Lincoln, Winston Churchill, and Edgar Allan Poe. Different in many ways, the one thing they shared, was knowledge of the Beast. Depression is not selective; it afflicts men and women, the young and the old, the rich and the poor.

Although Major Depression has existed across the centuries, it was long overlooked as a mental illness. Individuals with Major Depression are not usually dangerous or harmful to anyone ... with the exception of themselves. Physicians interested in diseases of the mind, focused their efforts toward the more obvious and potentially harmful (to others) disorders. Often someone's depression did not draw any attention until he or she committed suicide. Of course, by then it was too late.

Depression was commonly referred to as "the Melancholy" and numerous potions were devised to cure people of the Melancholy. These useless concoctions typically contained alcohol or laudanum and a lot people became addicted to what they hoped and prayed was a cure for their depression. Laudanum is a liquid containing several different opiates and was commonly used as a treatment for depression. Prominent literary figures such as Edgar Allan Poe, and John Keats[5] were believed to have used laudanum to escape their depression and provide them inspiration.

Many individuals with Major Depression were thought to be simply alcoholics or drug addicts and were shunned by society. Considered social outcasts, and avoided by those around them, these sad souls climbed further into their addiction and ceased interacting with anyone at all. Their tendency to isolate, and the inability to fight their addictions, only served to build the growing stereotypes society held against individuals suffering from Major Depression.

The biological origin of Major Depression was identified as early as 400 BC, when Hippocrates attributed depression to an excess of "black bile" in the system. Hippocrates described four temperaments he believed belonged to mankind: choleric, sanguine, melancholic, and phlegmatic.[6] He believed that human sickness resulted when the bodily fluids that were responsible for these temperaments became unbalanced. Black bile theory persisted well into the 1800s, and led to numerous treatments that attempted to bring these fluids back into balance.

When treatment was attempted, it often consisted of bleeding, applying leeches, inducing vomiting, and sweating out the poison that was causing the depression. It is probable that many depressives committed suicide in an attempt to escape the help of those who wished to cure them. Sometimes an individual with MDD would claim a miraculous recovery simply to avoid further treatment. Hiding our depression is not new; depressives have been hiding their illness for centuries.

The Suicide Connection

Historically, depression received the most attention when the individual committed suicide. Suicide victims were often buried in separate cemetery plots, or as was the custom in a few cultures, at a crossroads with a stake driven through the body.[7] The theory behind this bizarre custom was so it would be difficult for the deceased's ghost to escape the grave and find its way back to haunt the living. Most cultures frowned on suicide so heavily that they took every step possible to deny the suicide even happened. Denying that the suicide happened doesn't change the fact that it did.

Virtually every religion condemns the act of suicide. Many religious leaders taught that suicide victims were condemned to Hell or forced to roam the earth for eternity. Suicide victims were usually denied burial rites. More information on religious rites is discussed in Chapter 10. Family members were disgraced, often to the point of being shunned from the surrounding community. The stigma surrounding suicide was so overpowering, that frequently the coroner listed other causes of death to spare the family the ridicule and shame they would have been subjected to, were the suicide made public.

Modern suicide statistics report that suicide happens more often in recent years than in the past. Many experts debate whether social anxiety, pressures of modern living, or any number of other absurd ideas are the cause. I believe it isn't that suicides happen more frequently today, just that they are reported more accurately.

Depressives were often labeled as alcoholics and addicts in the past; frequently these deaths received little notice or attention. With suicide victims being condemned to Hell by the righteous, and family members shamed by the community, great effort was taken to call the death something else. In an attempt to spare the surviving family, many coroners and morticians took their secrets to the grave.

Depression Doesn't Begin to Describe the Beast

Is it any wonder individuals with depression don't want to tell anyone about the Beast? Ignorance, lack of compassion, and being judged, all lead depressives to hide their depression. The Beast loves to live in the darkness. Normal people sometimes ask the individual with Major Depression to describe what it feels like. There are no words to describe the Beast. Analogies such as living in the fog help normal individuals see a glimpse of what the depressive goes through. Calling what someone with MDD goes through as "depression" is a very poor description. Referring to the Beast as "depression" is an injustice to the Beast.

Chapter 3
The Creation of a Beast
Where Does Depression Come From?

People with MDD have many names for their depression. Two of the more common names are, "The Beast" and "The Black Dog"; I refer to my depression as simply my "Fog." The fact that some MDD individuals name their depression illustrates how much the disorder becomes a familiar and frequent companion.

Once depressives become familiar with their depression, they learn to recognize the signs when the Beast is planning another visit. Depression acts like an unwanted guest who refuses to leave and keeps coming back every time you think you've gotten rid of him. Naming our depression is a form of acceptance that the guest will continue to reappear for the rest of our lives.

Sometimes it feels incredibly unfair that I have this disease. To go through life knowing that at any time the Beast may reappear, is to live in constant anticipation of the next big storm. Sometimes it seems as if God is punishing me. I don't blame Him because I have this illness; I reconciled myself long ago that something as ugly as the Beast could never come from God. However, sometimes I feel as if God has turned a deaf ear to my prayers that I be allowed to die. Knowing the pain and loneliness of depression, I could never wish this madness on anyone. It is hard to understand how God can.

Winston Churchill called his depression his Black Dog[8] and often referred to his Black Dog returning to indicate he was once again sinking into the depths of his depression. For many people, the image of Churchill's snarling, black dog, slowly advancing with fangs bared, creates a perfect image of depression. Like a menacing dog preparing to strike, reasoning with depression is futile and we feel completely helpless to stop the approaching attack. Just as a mad dog silently circles its victim before closing in, depression patiently stalks its prey, and the individual with Major Depression reconciles him or herself to inevitable submission.

Discovering You're Not Alone

For the longest time, I believed I was completely alone; that the depression I felt, was something only I felt. Telling someone I was depressed usually resulted in a half-hearted attempt to "fix" me, or a poorly veiled annoyance with me for dampening everyone's mood. No one seemed to understand how I felt and this only reinforced my feelings of being alone. I believed there was something wrong with me and sensed I needed to hide it at all cost. When everyone else seems to be different, the only conclusion you can draw is that you are the one who is strange.

The first time I met another depressive I was thrilled to learn I wasn't the only one who had these kinds of thoughts. For the first time in my life I felt I had found someone with whom I could share my innermost thoughts and not be judged for them. She and I would talk until the early hours of the morning, baring our souls and sharing things we had never dared talk about with anyone before. We talked about the darkness, the hopelessness, and about our past suicide attempts. We talked about the burden of carrying our secret for so long, and how wonderful it was to finally find a kindred soul.

She had a cap gun that looked real (sort of), and individual caps could be loaded in the chambers and the barrel spun, just like an actual pistol. We would sometimes play Russian roulette with it and fantasize what it would be like to use a real gun. For this reason, I won't own a gun, and I frequently recommend to other depressives to get rid of their guns

I've learned over the years that this type of depressive bonding is very unhealthy, and should be placed on a list of activities to avoid at all costs. At the time I just focused on how good it felt to find another soul like me. I sometimes wonder if she is still alive, or if she ever got tired of using a cap gun and switched to a real one.

Over the years I have met many individuals with MDD. At first it was difficult to find them, however, as I began to recognize the same traits in others that I possessed myself, I became bolder about broaching the subject. Depressives become so conditioned to not talk about their depression, that bringing up the subject is very uncomfortable for them. I have been with people whom I strongly suspected were depressives, and have been afraid to say anything for fear they would think I was crazy, or worse, judge me for my own depression.

As I met one depressive after another, I began to realize that my condition was far more common than I had realized. At that time, the common label applied to my condition was "Clinical Depression." Although not a lot was known about Clinical Depression, doctors had at least determined it was the result of a biological condition. I was just grateful that it wasn't my imagination and that I wasn't crazy. The fog is overwhelming enough without questioning whether it is even real.

When I was 22, I met a doctor (the first of many) who told me I was clinically depressed. He scared me so bad I never went back. I realize now that I wasn't ready; at the time I was worried he was going to lock me up in a padded room and throw away the key.

He started talking about the different types of medications he could prescribe, and all I was able to think about were the stories I had heard that antidepressants could lead to suicidal thoughts. I knew I didn't need any help in that area; I had enough suicidal thoughts on my own. I put on my happy mask, tuned the doctor out, and left his office knowing fully that I would never return.

I do however owe that doctor my gratitude because he gave me a huge gift; he provided a name for my illness. Being a loner, I have always enjoyed doing research, and hearing the name "Clinical Depression," made me want to learn more. Where does Clinical Depression come from? Can Clinical Depression be treated? Is it curable? Who else has had clinical depression? At last the Beast had a face and a name. The more I learned about depression, the more I saw my reflection in what I read.

In Good Company

Individuals with Major Depression have a reputation for being very artistic. This shared talent or ability that's common among many depressives, is most probably traceable to brain development and overly active areas of the brain. A long-standing joke states that a child who appears depressed is going to grow up to be an artist; people often joke about things they don't understand. Differences in brain chemistry, and overly active areas of the brain are explained further in the next chapter. For now, suffice it to say that depressives are well known for their artistic talents.

Individuals with Major Depression often search for alternate ways to express themselves, to make their thoughts and feelings known to others. Simply stating they are "depressed" is misleading and does not begin to do justice to the Beast. Many depressives turn to whatever artistic medium they are best able to communicate through. Many well-known painters, sculptors, writers, and poets have been on intimate terms with the Beast. Many have died from the relationship.

One of the more notable writers to have been cursed with Major Depression was Ernest Hemingway. In 1929, he wrote in a letter to F. Scott Fitzgerald, "That terrible mood of depression of whether it is

any good or not, is what is known as the Artist's Reward."[9] Some
literary scholars today debate whether Hemingway even had Major
Depression, making the argument that a writer's life is conducive
to normal depression. I would argue that Major Depression lends
itself to a writer's life. Depressives tend to isolate, and they often
choose professions that allow them to work alone, such as writing.
I suspect that Hemingway would agree with me. In 1961 Hemingway
killed himself with his favorite shotgun.,

Virginia Woolf was another well-known author who experienced
Major Depression. Today she would probably be diagnosed with
bipolar disorder (very similar to Major Depression). She frequently
spoke of, and wrote about, her depression in her diaries.[10] Woolf had
numerous severe episodes of depression throughout her life and
often referred to them as her "Madness." After several failed suicide
attempts, she finally completed suicide in 1941 when she filled
her pockets with rocks, and drowned herself in a river behind her
home.

The list goes on and on. I have found comfort in knowing that
I'm not alone; that others share my knowledge of the fog. It makes
the world seem like a less lonely place. Reading the words of
another depressive allows me to bond with the writer, because I
know what he or she is feeling. Viewing a painting or a sculpture
by someone with Major Depression, provides me the opportunity
to experience that person's pain and despair, knowing their art is
the depressive's attempt to hold onto his or her sanity. Having a

common enemy allows depressives to support each other in a way no one else can. In the words of the poet John Donne (another depressive), "Each man's death diminishes me, for I am involved in mankind."

It's ironic that individuals with a disorder that makes them seek isolation, find comfort in the company of others with the same disorder, and preference for being alone. Individuals with Major Depression become so accustomed to hiding their depression, that the freedom afforded them from not having to maintain their secret is liberating. The shared familiarity of the Beast affords an opportunity for depressives to let down their hair and no longer feel the need to gauge each other's reaction after every sentence is spoken. Reading the words of depressive writers or viewing the work of depressive artists creates a kinship through compassion for the writer or artist's pain.

I have heard countless individuals state they believe having depression makes a person a better writer or a better artist. The tone of some non-depressed writers is almost one of envy or covetousness. What they don't realize, or choose to forget, are the long periods of darkness and despair where the depressive is often unable even to get up out of bed, never mind being able to sit at a keyboard and bleed out their thoughts.

During Virginia Woolf's worst depressive episodes she was unable to care for herself, and she could not write a sensible word. Hemingway had long streaks where he was unable to write a thing.

During Edgar Allan Poe's most severe depression he roamed the streets aimlessly, in a drunken and drug-induced stupor. Although many depressives are highly artistic, the talent does not come from their depression, it comes from deep inside them. If anything, the depression hinders them from being even better.

Where Does Major Depression Come From?

The cause behind Major Depression is hotly debated among psychology professionals; they can't seem to agree where it comes from. One thing they do agree on is that Major Depression is largely hereditary. If you've ever seen a medical questionnaire with the question, "Is there a history of suicide in your family?" that's the reason why. The physician or therapist is interested in whether there is a genetic history of Major Depression in your family. Because depressives often hide their disorder from friends and loved ones, asking about suicide provides a much clearer picture of a genetic history.

You may be asking yourself, "If Major Depression is hereditary, why do some siblings appear to have it while others don't?" One popular theory is that Major Depression requires two things before the Beast can make its first appearance: 1) a predisposition toward Major Depression, 2) a triggering event. Is it possible for someone without a genetic predisposition to still develop Major Depression? In my opinion it is, however, because talking about depression was taboo in the past, and it was frequently kept a secret, it can be difficult to know whether Major Depression was present among someone's ancestors.

A more helpful use of genetic history, is when family depression is known to exist. This can be a good indicator that an individual has a predisposition toward depression. If a parent was depressed, even if he or she was never diagnosed with clinical depression, there is a strong likelihood the children will have a predisposition toward depression. If any family members are known to have committed suicide, the likelihood increases even further.

Just because an individual has a predisposition toward Major Depression does not ensure he or she will meet the Beast. Many families have one parent and one child who are depressives, while the remaining children never develop the disorder. Having a genetic predisposition toward Major Depression, also called a diathesis, simply means the individual is more likely to develop the disorder than someone who does not have the same predisposition.

Those who eventually develop the disorder, do so at different stages in their lives. My depression first peeked over the horizon at age 11, however I have known many depressives who did not experience their first episode until their 20s and a few who first showed signs of Major Depression in their 30s and 40s.

Having a predisposition toward Major Depression is like living with a bomb and waiting for someone to come along and light the fuse. The lighting of the fuse is what psychologists refer to as the "triggering event." Those with a predisposition toward MDD yet never developed the disorder, are fortunate enough to have never met someone with a match.

Triggering Events

As mentioned previously, having a predisposition toward Major Depression is not by itself sufficient to bring out the disorder; a triggering event is also required. A triggering event is something that happens that causes something else to happen. In the case of Major Depression, something happens that causes the individual to develop Major Depressive Disorder. Think of the predisposition as the Beast quietly hibernating inside the depressive. The triggering event is something that wakes the Beast up.

Triggering events vary from individual-to-individual. The person may experience something severe, such as a near fatal accident, or the triggering event may be something more innocuous such as being laughed at by a pretty girl or an attractive boy. One thing is certain: the triggering event is not retractable, you can't un-ring the bell. Once triggered, developing the depression disorder is inevitable. My triggering event was most likely my grandmother's suicide when I was 11. Even though I did not immediately fall into a depressive episode, something changed in me that day, and there was no returning to my former self.

Not everyone who is triggered, realizes it at the time. In therapy, a common exercise is to have the individual with Major Depression try to remember the first time he or she became depressed, or started feeling different. The point is to look for events that occurred around the same time that may have acted as the trigger. Although identifying the trigger helps the individual understand where his or her depression came from, it does not cure or reverse the person's depression. There is no going back.

Triggering events explain why multiple siblings can have the same parents and yet one sibling develops Major Depression while the others do not. Triggering events also offer an explanation why someone may appear normal and at one point in his or her life, and later show signs of Major Depression. In both cases, the depressives experienced an event that woke up the Beast within them.

How Do You Know If You Have It?

Having read this far, many individuals may be inclined to self-diagnose themselves with Major Depression. I cannot emphasize enough how bad of an idea this is. To begin with, there are similar disorders, such as bipolar disorder or post-partum depression, that share some common symptoms, however are treated differently. Secondly, as mentioned previously, everyone gets depressed at different times in his or her life. How do you distinguish between normal depression and Major Depression?

Professional psychologists use a guide named the DSM-5 when diagnosing someone with Major Depressive Disorder. This book is basically the mental health bible, and before anyone is diagnosed with a mental health disorder, he or she should first meet minimum criteria as stated in the DSM-5. Each mental health disorder is assigned an identifying code; the codes used for Major Depressive Disorder is F33.x; the x is a number dependent on the severity of the MDD.

The following criteria are used by the DSM-5 and can serve as a guide to whether individuals should seek professional help for their depression.

Five or more of the following symptoms must occur during a consecutive two-week period and must include at least one of the first two criteria:

(1) *Depressed mood most of the day, nearly every day, as appears by personal report or observation by others.*

(2) *Markedly diminished interest or pleasure in all, or almost all, activities most of the day, nearly every day.*

(3) *Significant weight loss when not dieting or weight gain, or decrease or increase in appetite nearly every day.*

(4) *Insomnia or hypersomnia nearly every day.*

(5) *Psychomotor agitation or retardation nearly every day.*

(6) *Fatigue or loss of energy nearly every day.*

(7) *Feelings of worthlessness or excessive or inappropriate guilt nearly every day.*

(8) *Diminished ability to think or concentrate, or indecisiveness, nearly every day.*

(9)   *Recurrent thoughts of death, recurrent suicidal ideation without a specific plan, or a suicide attempt or a specific plan for committing suicide.*

Feelings of worthlessness and suicide ideation are discussed further in Chapters 5 and 6. Many depressives easily meet seven, eight, and sometimes all nine criteria from the DSM-5. Individuals with normal depression neither meet that many criteria nor do they experience depression symptoms for the extended periods of time that depressives do. If after you read this list you feel you might have Major Depression, I highly recommend you see a professional who **specializes in Major Depressive Disorder** for a professional evaluation. I sometimes wonder what the Beast thinks of the list.

This Page left Intentionally Blank

Chapter 4
A Ticking Time Bomb
Inheriting More Than Good Looks

Life is unpredictable. At any moment, you could have a heart attack, be hit by a car, or have a meteorite fall on your head. It is the uncertainty with which we all live. Most people accept that they will one day die, and they hope it won't happen tomorrow. Some people live with the reality that it may very well happen soon, or at the very least, they will wish they were dead. This is the curse that depressives live with their entire lives. It's like living in Tornado Alley in the Midwest and waiting for the next storm to come. It's not a question of whether another storm will come, only when it will happen.

One universally accepted fact about Major Depression is that it is heritable; you get it from your parents. Not everyone who has a depressive parent will themselves develop MDD, however there is a reasonable probability that the individual will at least carry the gene. If both parents have depression in their family trees, the probability increases further. If neither of your parents suffer from depression does that mean you're safe? It doesn't. You would still need to look back to your grandparents, your great-grandparents, your crazy second-cousin Billy, twice removed on your great-grandmother's side of the family, etc.

Geneticists have identified the 5-HTT transporter gene as one of the genes involved in depressive disorders, however its role is not completely understood. Many mental health professionals argue that there are additional genes that haven't been identified yet that also increase the likelihood an individual will develop Major Depressive Disorder.[11] Some substance abuse professionals argue that the depression gene is different from the alcoholism gene, others argue it is the same.[12]

I am a substance abuse professional. I'm also a depression counselor, and I lean toward the theory that Major Depression and alcoholism both come from the same gene, or genes. We know beyond a doubt that the two are related because of the high co-occurrence of MDD in alcoholics (and vice versa). What this means to anyone with Major Depression is, 'stay away from alcohol' as you most likely have a genetic predisposition toward alcoholism. Alcohol and depression make a bad combination; depressives should not drink. For more information about the link between alcoholism and depression see Chapter 7.

The Role of Neurotransmitters

Think of Neurotransmitters as the brain's mailmen, passing letters from one nerve cell to the next. There are several types of neurotransmitters, and each is responsible for delivering a different type of message. When most people think of nerves, they associate them with pain or tremors, however nerves are responsible for all types of communication. Nerve signals are tied to: happiness, sadness, pleasure, depression, movement, temperature, sight, and anything else you can think of that requires one part of the body to communicate with another. If you have a feeling, emotion, or thought, you can be assured that neurotransmitters were involved.

When there are not enough neurotransmitters, the messages get backed up and not all the letters get delivered. When there are too many neurotransmitters, the messages flood the receiving cell and the person becomes overwhelmed. Fortunately, (and sometimes unfortunately), we have learned how to increase and decrease specific neurotransmitters to our advantage.

Positive uses for controlling neurotransmitters include: pain killers to block or decrease pain signals, medication to control the shaking associated with Parkinson's disease, and antidepressants for managing depression. Negative uses include the use of illegal drugs such as: cocaine, methamphetamines, and heroin. These drugs create of flood of neurotransmitters in the brain that can lead to high risk behavior, dependence, and addiction.

Serotonin is Our Friend

The neurotransmitter serotonin is the common one associated with depression, although there are several other neurotransmitters that play a role as well. Think of serotonin as the 'well-being' or 'feel normal' chemical. When you have enough serotonin you feel content, self-confident, and for the most part, you feel happy. When you don't have enough serotonin, you feel off or different from everyone else, you feel blue, and just generally 'blah.' You also lack the desire to do much of anything. Serotonin also plays a role in cardiovascular regulation, appetite, sexual desire, mood, anxiety, substance abuse, sleep, poor impulse control, and aggression to name just a few of its functions. Sufficient serotonin is very important in healthy living.

People with low serotonin are more prone to depression. They tend to feel worthless and hopeless. They lack self-confidence. Low serotonin levels also can make an individual feel more aggressive; many men suffering from depression are misdiagnosed as having anger problems.[13]

Poor impulse control is another common feature common with low serotonin, and often results in the individual being more likely to take part in high risk behaviors.[13] Substance abuse, particularly alcohol, is associated with serotonin deficiency; many individuals suffering from low serotonin, drink alcohol or take drugs to self-medicate the effects of serotonin deficiency. Low serotonin can also create carbohydrate cravings; food is another way people self-medicate.

Substances that Produce Serotonin

Unfortunately, you can't just take a serotonin pill; no such thing exists. Serotonin doesn't occur naturally in foods; it is a chemical our body makes from an amino acid called Tryptophan.[14] If you want to increase your serotonin level without medication, you need to increase your intake of tryptophan. Although serotonin isn't found in food, tryptophan is. Selling serotonin supplements is most likely just peddling tryptophan pills.

Foods that are high in tryptophan include: egg yolks, cheese, pineapples, bananas, all meats (not just turkey), nuts, green tea, and dark chocolate (the darker the better). It would be great if a diet of just these foods would relieve our depression; unfortunately, it's not that simple. We cannot live on chocolate alone; tryptophan heavy foods need some help.

To help your body absorb tryptophan, you'll need to use the carb connection. Dieticians may tell you that carbohydrates are bad; however, your mental health professional will tell you that carbohydrates are a necessary part of a healthy serotonin diet.[15] Carbohydrates, such as potatoes, pasta, and white breads help your body absorb more tryptophan, which will in turn make more serotonin. It's best to eat small amounts of carbs throughout the day to maximize your absorption of tryptophan.

An ideal serotonin diet consists of small amounts of carbs along with tryptophan rich foods. Sounds like comfort food, doesn't it? It is. Now you know why you feel better after eating steak and potatoes for dinner, and dark chocolate cake for dessert. A good depression diet includes eating at least one tryptophan heavy food during every meal, and small amounts of carbs throughout the day.

The third ingredient required in serotonin production is vitamin D. Sunshine is probably the best way to increase your vitamin D levels, because when sunlight strikes your skin, you produce your own vitamin D. Vitamin D turn regulates the conversion of tryptophan into serotonin. Spending 10-20 minutes a day outside in the sun (with exposed skin), will do wonders for your depression. Please be aware that excessive exposure to sunlight can lead to skin cancer. It must also be noted that the darker your skin is, the less vitamin D is produced, therefore individuals with darker skin need to stay in the sun longer to achieve the same effect.[16]

As an alternative to laying in the sun, D-3 supplements can also provide the same effect. These vitamins are sold in strengths ranging from 400 IU to 5000 IU. For someone who has normal serotonin levels, the lower doses are fine for maintenance. However, if you have a serotonin deficiency, these lower dosages won't do you much good and you will need to use one of the higher dosages. Studies have shown that vitamin D supplements don't start showing an effect on depression levels until at least 4000 IU.[16] Always consult with your Doctor before adding any daily supplement to your diet to ensure there will be no conflicts with any prescription medications you may be taking.

Antidepressants

There are many classifications of prescription antidepressants including: MAOIs, TCAs, SSRIs, SNRIs, and Atypicals. Each of these classifications has several different medications. The most popular anti-depressants in the last 10-20 years are SSRIs and SNRIs, and for good reason, they have fewer side effects. This is not to say these medications are free of side effects, they are just more easily tolerated by most people.

SSRI stands for Selective Serotonin Reuptake Inhibitor. These medications make you nerve cells hold on to serotonin longer before it is reabsorbed. Although these medications do not create more serotonin, keeping the little serotonin you have longer, essentially accomplishes the same thing. SSRIs include: fluoxetine (Prozac), sertraline (Zoloft), fluvoxamine (Luvox), paroxetine (Paxil, Pexeva), citalopram (Celexa), and escitalopram (Lexapro).[17] Not everyone responds to every SSRI the same, so your doctor may have to try a couple different ones before you find one that works.

SNRIs are similar to SSRIs ... only different. SNRI stands for Serotonin Norepinephrine Reuptake Inhibitors. Whereas SSRIs only affect serotonin levels, SNRIs also affect a neurotransmitter called norepinephrine. Norepinephrine is associated with arousal and energy. It could be said that an SNRI is a neurotransmitter cocktail in which the negative effects of the serotonin reuptake inhibitor are partially offset for by the positive effects of the norepinephrine reuptake inhibitor. Stated simply, SNRIs have fewer side effects than SSRIs. SNRIs include: venlafaxine (Effexor), desvenlafaxine (Pristiq, Khedezia), and duloxetine (Cymbalta).[17]

Although on the surface it may seem like SNRIs are a better choice than SSRIs for treating depression, however not everyone responds the same to them. Additionally, if an individual suffers from bipolar disorder, some SNRIs have been known to bring on mania episodes.[17] Sometimes an SSRI is the best medication to take; always work with your doctor in choosing an appropriate medication for you.

Bupropion (Wellbutrin) is an antidepressant that stands by itself. This medication is referred to as an Atypical, which simply means it doesn't fit into any of the other classifications. Bupropion doesn't affect serotonin levels, instead it inhibits the reuptake of dopamine and norepinephrine.[17] Simply said, bupropion increases the amount of dopamine and norepinephrine in the brain. Bupropion is often prescribed to augment an SSRI medication.

There are many reasons to take bupropion, some of which include: no sexual side effects (some people report an increase in sexual desire), dampening of situational depression, and increased energy.[17] Essentially, bupropion can counteract many of the side effects from SSRI medications, and treat several of the symptoms associated with Major Depression.

Abilify is a supplemental drug for treating depression; it is taken along with an antidepressant to improve its performance. Abilify acts by increasing dopamine levels when they are low; the drug effectively makes antidepressant (and bipolar) medications work better.[17] If after taking this drug you notice a significant increase in the amount of time you are sleeping, please notify your doctor immediately.

When You Have a Headache, You Take Aspirin

The negative stigma surrounding depression is so great that many individuals who suffer from Major Depression, are afraid to take antidepressant medication. These individuals may believe taking medication makes them appear weak, or they may be afraid of how they will react to the drugs. Using homeopathic treatments such as serotonin diets and vitamin D supplements are great, but for many people, there is a point where the natural approach simply isn't enough.

Some individuals are frightened of antidepressants because of the warning labels, "May cause suicidal thoughts in children." There is considerable debate in the mental health fields on whether this is even accurate, however even those professionals who believe the warning is appropriate, admit that such cases are rare. If this is a concern of yours then ask a close friend to keep an eye on you, and if you find yourself having suicidal thoughts, confide in your friend, or your doctor, or both. Close monitoring for four to six weeks is normal for anyone starting on antidepressants.

The bottom line is this: if you suffer from Major Depression, antidepressants will probably help you feel better. When someone has a headache he or she takes an aspirin, when an individual has diabetes, using diabetes medication is a no brainer, and when a person is diagnosed with cancer the doctor places him or her on chemotherapy. Ironically, when many people feel depressed and worthless, they resist taking the medication that will make them feel better.

A more common problem, is people who take their prescribed antidepressants, start feeling better, and then stop taking their antidepressants because they are feeling better. The individual was feeling better BECAUSE he or she was taking the antidepressant to begin with. Always follow your doctor's advice when you are taking antidepressants, and even more importantly, when discontinuing them. Suddenly stopping your antidepressant medication on your own can be dangerous; follow your doctor's guidelines.

Medication Is Not Evil

There are many things in this world that simply should not be. Headlines in the news bring the most recent tragedy to our fingertips every morning. People are starving in the slums just miles from where others waste enough food to feed a family of four for a week. Violence perpetrated by children erupts in our schools. Medication should not be counted among the world's evils. We are fortunate to live during a time when antidepressant medications are available. A mere 75 years ago, depressives had no choice but to suffer in silence; today we have options.

If you choose to use the more natural methods to treat your depression, that is your choice; I chose to do the same for many years. Please make no mistake though, these methods are not a substitute for medication, and will not work as well. Because of antidepressant medication, you no longer must suffer the pain from depression without any relief; when you have a headache you take an aspirin don't you?

This Page left Intentionally Blank

Chapter 5
A Life Without Value
Worthlessness as a Way of Life

As long as I can remember, I have hated my birthday. Family members buying gifts, surprise parties, everyone pretending they cared about my birthday; who did they think they were kidding? People with Major Depression hate being made a fuss over for the simple reason, we don't believe we're worthy of the attention. Being unworthy frequently extends into every area of a depressive's life. Reluctance to buy clothes (or anything else), is a trait shared by many depressives. Letting someone else choose the restaurant, always letting others go first, and denying ourselves the simplest pleasures becomes a way life for individuals with MDD.

Low Self-Esteem

Self-esteem refers to how someone thinks about him or herself. Individuals with high self-esteem see themselves in a positive light; people with low self-esteem think less of themselves. Individuals with MDD tend to think very little of themselves and have a very poor self-image. Many psychologists believe that low self-esteem results from a lack of supporting relationships during childhood, especially relationships with parents or guardians.[18] Depressives know our low self-esteem comes from the Beast. Our depression lies to us, it tricks us, and it saps our strength to the point that we are too weak

63

to argue. For many people suffering from Major Depression, low self-esteem is the only thing they've ever known.

How low someone's self-esteem drops, is largely a matter of how much depression he or she is experiencing. The higher an individual's depression climbs, the lower his or her self-esteem will fall. Tumbling self-esteem often becomes apparent through poor hygiene or grooming; when people experience low self-esteem, they are less likely to care about their outward appearances. A depressed person may skip bathing, cease shaving, or stop using makeup. Likewise, he or she may choose unflattering clothes, may no longer wear clean clothes, or may stop getting dressed in the morning altogether.

What can someone with Major Depression do about their low self-esteem? To begin with, it's essential we admit our low self-esteem is unhealthy. I've never met a person who actually enjoyed his or her low self-esteem. Recognize low self-esteem for what it is, a tool the Beast uses to hold us down. Secondly, realize that self-esteem does not come from others; it comes from inside us. Building self-esteem doesn't just happen; it takes personal effort. It's our choice whether or not to put forth that effort.

No matter how much we don't want to, we need to maintain our personal appearance as if nothing was wrong. When we allow our personal hygiene to slip, it drives our self-esteem lower. When our self-esteem drops, we stop caring about our appearance. It becomes a vicious cycle, and like a rolling snowball, it grows larger the longer it continues. Resisting our depression, by maintaining our personal appearance, is also a choice.

Hating Compliments

When someone gives me a compliment, the first thing I feel is resentment. How dare that person say something we both know isn't true? I immediately assume the other individual must want something; why else would he or she be saying that? People with Major Depression hate compliments. If you want to start an argument with a depressive, give him or her a compliment. We'll tell you all the reasons we don't deserve it. Given the option, most depressives would endure a hurricane to avoid a compliment.

You may be thinking, "Lots of people hate compliments." The difference between a normal person and an individual with MDD, is his or her self-acknowledgment of their accomplishment. When normal people receive compliments, they may feel embarrassed or uncomfortable. They may also be shy and wish to avoid any personal attention. They may, or may not, feel a sense of pride for their accomplishment. It is the praise that makes them uncomfortable. Normal people accomplish things, and the pride they feel varies depending on the value they place on the achievement.

When a person with MDD receives a compliment, he or she usually assumes it is a false compliment and mentally discredits it. It isn't shyness, but rather disbelief, that prevents someone with Major Depression from accepting compliments. Individuals with MDD have a difficult time seeing their achievements as accomplishments. Most individuals with Major Depression either receive no pride from their accomplishments, or if they do, it is short-lived and lasts no more than a few hours. Many people close to me have said I should be proud of the things I have accomplished in my life; I tell them I don't even know what that feels like.

How should someone with MDD handle compliments? Give the other person the benefit of the doubt that he or she is sincere. Even if we don't believe we're worthy of the compliment, we need to remember that our thoughts can't always be trusted. Compliments affect both the person giving it and the one receiving. Accepting a compliment, even when we don't believe it, is a reminder our depression also affects those around us. Whether we realize it or not, receiving a compliment has a positive effect on us and we need all the positives we can get.

The Cloak of Invisibility

Since the first time I heard of a cloak of invisibility, I have been fascinated with the concept. Even though the garment is pure fiction, the very idea captures my imagination and sends it racing. Imagine being able to move around other people without being seen? No more having to hide in the house behind closed curtains. No longer waiting until it's dark to go to the store. It's a depressive's dream. Learning to be invisible without a cloak can takes years of practice.

Individuals with Major Depression typically dislike crowds and avoid them whenever possible. Crowds don't feel safe. When I am in a depressive episode, the last thing I want is to be around people. Many depressives experience periods of agoraphobia (fear of crowds and being trapped) when they are having an episode. Just the thought of a crowded store can be enough to trigger a panic attack. The desire to close all the curtains, and not step outside until the storm has passed, can be overwhelming.

In the late 70s there was a sitcom named *Soap* in which one of the characters (Bert) thought he had the power to make himself invisible. Whenever he felt uncomfortable or afraid, he waved his hands and snapped his fingers to make himself disappear (so he thought). Anyone with MDD will recognize this character as a fellow depressive. If I had been him, I would have remained invisible all the time.

We spend years perfecting our powers of invisibility. Learning to fade into the background when in a group, dressing plainly so as not to stand out, keeping our opinions to ourselves, are all skills required to be a successful depressive. Invisibility is a depressive's favorite survival skill; the alternative is for individuals with MDD to be noticed for who they really are. The Beast is cunning; becoming invisible doesn't happen all at once. Someone with Major Depression doesn't wake up one day and decide that he or she is going to disappear. It happens slowly over time; like the approaching fog. As the discomfort around others increases, individuals with MDD fade further and further away.

The worst part about being invisible is that when you're hurting, no one can find you to help. When someone is lost in a depressive episode, that person needs to be around others more than ever. However, the Beast convinces us to hide, to stay indoors, and to become invisible. When someone feels the fog closing in, that person desperately needs to feel the warmth of the sun on his or her face. Unfortunately, that is when the Beast tells the depressive to hide indoors with the curtains closed. Fighting the urge to be invisible means getting out in the daylight, and around other people, even when it's the last thing you feel like doing. Taking off the cloak of invisibility is difficult, but it can be done.

What is Value?

When people value something, they show a preference toward it. Given the choice between object A and object B, they will always pick the object they value the most. What is of value to one person may not be to another; it all comes down to individual preference. When given a choice between chocolate cake and Brussel sprouts, I personally will always value the chocolate cake more.

What does it mean therefore, to have "A Life Without Value?" Does it refer to other people's preference for non-depressives, or does it refer to an individual's self-perception? Depending on the circumstances, some people may receive a higher preference in another's eyes; some are given a lower one. Anyone who has ever been picked last to play on a team knows the embarrassment of being assigned a lower value. Any "normal person" who has ever come in first place, knows the pride of being assigned a higher value. Whether referring to home prices, someone's salary, or who will win the next Super Bowl, assigning value is part of life.

Individuals with MDD tend to believe no one would prefer them over someone else. We expect to be picked last for the team. If it doesn't happen, it's because (we assume) the other person feels sorry for us. If we do something important and worthy of praise, we wait for the feeling of pride to come; it rarely does. Winning always seems anti-climactic. Success is tempered by the feeling, "there should be more." Others have told us what it feels like to be proud and the emotion seems to forever escape us.

People with Major Depression assume no one places value on them because they place no value in themselves. When every day is filled with emotional pain, from the moment someone wakes up, until he or she falls asleep, not waking up begins to have more value than its alternative. Some individuals with MDD discover they prefer death to living; at that point, they have come to a dark and dangerous crossroad. Suicide is discussed more in Chapter 6, for now suffice it to say that believing death has a higher value than life can be the first step in suicide's direction.

Never Good Enough

Many people with Major Depression are also perfectionists. It's not that we insist on doing something perfectly; it's just that no matter how well we do a job, it's never good enough. Individuals with MDD are hard on themselves; the Beast tells us to do it. When we fail at something, no matter how trivial, we insist on beating ourselves up over it. If someone tells us he or she is disappointed in us, we flog ourselves mercilessly, sometimes for days or weeks. Our depression not only tells us we're not good enough; it has the audacity to say we never will be. The Beast is very cruel.

When I find myself sinking once again into the pit, telling myself that's where I belong, I sometimes wonder if Hemingway or Poe ever came to believe they were good enough. Did they finally reach a point where they deemed themselves worthy? Personally, I doubt it; depression is like that. It sometimes feels like my depression is a curse; a leech that sucks the life from me, and like all parasites, it gives nothing in return.

Like others with low self-esteem, individuals with MDD tend to put themselves down in front of others. We call ourselves names like stupid, idiot, and jerk as if we were talking about the weather. I've heard normal people say they think we put ourselves down so someone will disagree with us. Quite the opposite is true, we hope no one will say a word and therefore confirm the statement with their silence. It is far easier for individuals with MDD to say something bad about themselves than something good.

The problem with putting ourselves down, is that negative talk begets more negative talk, and self-deprecation feeds the Beast and makes it stronger. Although I am the first to admit it's difficult, it is nevertheless extremely important for depressives to resist the urge to put themselves down. Just as putting ourselves down is a choice we make, not verbalizing negative comments is "also" a conscious choice.

Inappropriate Guilt

If someone I love is feeling down, I know beyond a doubt it's my fault. Whenever something bad happens to anyone near me, it's because I caused it. If a natural disaster happens on the other side of the world, somehow, I'll find a way to take the blame for that too. People with Major Depression have a talent for finding ways to assume guilt for each misfortune, any calamity, and every failure around them. If it weren't so sad it would be comical.

It's bad enough that depressives want to assume the blame for everything around them, but they also often apologize for things they didn't do. If a family member injures him or herself, we're right there saying how sorry we are. When a child gets a bad grade, we ask for forgiveness for not helping him or her study more. When a spouse has his or her favorite television show pre-empted for a presidential address, we apologize for that too. I imagine this habit has got to drive normal people nuts.

According to the DSM-5, the symptoms used to diagnose MDD include, "Feelings of worthlessness or excessive or inappropriate guilt nearly every day." I always knew my feelings of worthlessness and guilt weren't normal. What I didn't realize for the longest time, was that there were others like me who felt the same way. When I realized other depressives shared these same feelings, I felt less like a freak. The Beast tells us no one will understand and convinces us to remain silent; learning there are others who think and feel the same way can be liberating.

When people assume blame for things they didn't do, therapists call it "irrational thinking." It's obvious (even to the depressive) that no one is responsible for the presidential address (except maybe the president), or a natural disaster on the other side of the world. Part of a therapist's job is to challenge these irrational thoughts and help the MDD individual replace them with more rational ones. Failure to challenge an irrational thought, only serves to reinforce it through silence.

Living with Major Depressive Disorder requires us to challenge our thoughts whenever they seem suspicious. Recognizing that our thoughts cannot be trusted is a major step in the right direction. Using someone as a sounding board can provide us a levelheaded perspective. I have learned to use my wife to bounce off thoughts I'm uncertain about. When a thought doesn't feel right, or I suspect it might be my depression talking, I share my thoughts with my wife, and she lets me know when my depression is lying to me again.

72

Developing this kind of trust relationship with someone can take time and practice, however it is a very crucial coping skill.

Blowing Our Own Horn

An old idiom says, "If you don't blow your own horn, no one will blow it for you." Living with Major Depression is like fighting a life-long war. Each depressive episode is the equivalent of a new battle, and like any well-trained military, we need to prepare ahead for those battles during peacetime. Blowing our own horn simply means we take credit for our accomplishments, and inform others about them.

Taking credit for our achievements when we are between episodes, builds self-esteem, acknowledges we have value, and prepares us for the next visit by the Beast. Letting our supervisor know we finished ahead of schedule, informing our spouse we lost another two pounds on our diet, and telling an acquaintance we achieved a goal are all examples of blowing our own horn.

The problem with the cloak of invisibility is that no one can see us. Of course, that's the whole point, however it means the individual with Major Depression gets passed up for promotions, gets overlooked by potential mates, and in general, misses out on a great deal of life. Just because individuals with MDD don't assert themselves or seek to be noticed, doesn't mean they don't desire promotions as much as the next person. As much as people with

MDD don't want to, blowing their own horns is essential to managing Major Depression and surviving life.

Sometimes I get so tired of my depression that I want to scream. I hate what it has done to my life, and I hate what it has stolen from me. Just once, I would like to accomplish something and feel pride well up inside me. Just once, I would like someone to tell me "great job" and not feel the urge to argue with them. Mostly, I would like to know what it feels like to be "normal." These are just a few of the things my depression has robbed me of.

I wish I could tell you to drink lots of vitamin C, or meditate for fifteen minutes every morning and your Major Depression will go away; but I can't, because it won't. Take a walk down any self-help aisle of a local bookstore and the shelves are filled with books that tell you how to "cure your depression." In the author's pictures on the back-jacket cover, they always look so incredibly happy; it makes me nauseous every time I see them.

Our Depression is relentless; we must behave the same way in return. As explained previously in Chapter 4, Major Depression has biological roots. Taking a pill doesn't make depression go away, and neither does blowing your own horn. However, what taking an antidepressant, or blowing your own horn does accomplish, is to push the Beast further back.

The war against depression isn't won in a single battle, but in a series of skirmishes that keep the enemy at bay. Blowing our own horn is just another one of the tools in our arsenal. Every time we push the Beast back, we are taking action to ensure our survival. The Beast would like us to lay down and give up, blowing our own horn says we refuse to let our depression win.

This Page left Intentionally Blank

Chapter 6
Keys to the Prison
No Other Way Out

John Donne wrote, "Whenever my affliction assails me, methinks I have the keys of my prison in my own hand, and no remedy presents itself so soon to my heart as mine own sword.[19]" Donne was obviously a depressive; his words echo the thoughts of every depressive who has ever contemplated suicide. Comparing Major Depression to a prison is a metaphor that even non-depressives can understand. Comparing suicide to the keys is a comparison that will challenge the values of most people who read this.

Major Depression absolutely feels like a prison, and for many people it's a life-sentence. The lucky individuals whose depression is in remission, know they could be locked up again at any time. The worst part about being in prison is the total loss of control; all your decisions are made for you. The Beast is our jail-keeper, relentlessly watching over us and preventing us from joining our loved ones and the life we long to have. It sometimes feels as if I am watching the world through steel bars, tormented by what is just beyond my reach.

When someone asks me, "What drives a person to attempt suicide?", I tell the person, "hopelessness." Normies mistakenly think when someone attempts suicide it is because the individual wants to die. Most people don't commit suicide because they want to die; they do it because they want the pain to stop. Given the choice between living happily ever after and dying, the clear majority of depressives would choose to live their dreams.

Sadly, for many depressives those dreams come to resemble unicorns and fairy tales; childhood fantasies that hold no basis in reality. The Fog has a way of obscuring our dreams. One by one, our dreams of happiness and success disappear, until all we have left is total isolation with no hope of ever finding our way back. Hopelessness is the absence of hope. To be hopeless means there is no remedy or cure; no chance of the situation ever improving. Hopelessness is one of the defining symptoms of Major Depressive Disorder. Hopelessness is also the primary reason that people commit suicide.

Hopelessness led me toward that cliff when I was seventeen. It was also responsible for my filling up a bathtub and reaching for the hair dryer when I was twenty-seven. Hopelessness has killed more people than all the wars in the history of mankind combined. When problems become overwhelming, it can feel like there is no way out, no possible solution. When no solution is apparent, that person enters the dark room of hopelessness. Should the thought of suicide occur, it can suddenly seem like a light at the end of the tunnel, an open door through which escape is possible. People who have never been suicidal frequently ask why someone makes the choice to take his or her life; it's because the suicidal individual believes there is no other way out.

Depression and Suicide

It's estimated that up to 70% of individuals who commit suicide are having a depressive episode at the time of their death; obviously, there is a connection between the two.[19] In the United States alone there are over 43,000 suicides every year, and over 25,000 of these individuals suffered from Major Depression.[20] That equates to 20,000 suicide fatalities (80%) every year who never even sought treatment for their depression. These statistics don't even begin to consider the attempts that weren't completed. Considering that Major Depression is treatable, that's a lot of people who had other options and didn't even realize it.

Major Depression often remains undiagnosed. It's estimated that up to 80% of individuals who have MDD are undiagnosed and will never seek treatment. These poor souls often take their secret to the grave; and because of their depression, that trip sometimes occurs sooner instead of later. The exact number of suicides resulting from depression is unknown because many unnatural deaths, such as head-on car crashes and drug overdoses, are also thought to be suicides. There is no way to know for certain how many of these deaths were planned, because only 20 percent of suicide victims leave notes confirming their intentions.[19]

Considering the large number of undiagnosed people with Major Depression, is it any wonder that so many suicides leave loved ones painfully shocked; oblivious that a problem even existed? The need for secrecy, and the depressive's ability to put on a "happy mask," often leaves family members completely unaware of the individual's illness until after he or she has committed suicide. Family members are frequently left questioning each other about what went wrong; many loved ones blame themselves for not having seen the signs. These individuals should not assume blame; the reason they didn't see the signs is because the suicidal individual was good at hiding his or her depression.

Suicide and Major Depression are so closely linked together that a history of suicide attempts is considered one of the strongest indicators of Major Depressive Disorder. A previous suicide attempt is also considered to be the leading risk factor for future attempts. Many psychologists speculate why this is true; my belief is that once an individual has mentally gone to that dark place, it's easier to find his or her way back.

Suicide is also used as the primary indicator of a family history of Depression. Because of the social stigmas associated with Major Depression, and the fact that such a large percentage of cases go undiagnosed, establishing a family predisposition toward depression can be difficult. Many medical professionals turn to a family history of suicide when looking for evidence of Major Depressive Disorder. Most medical intake forms ask if anyone in the family has ever committed suicide. Medical professionals used to believe the very act of suicide itself was heritable and a few still subscribe to this theory. My belief is that suicide is the behavior and outcome of Major Depression; it's not the disease.

Disappearing Act

Children enjoy playing in large cardboard boxes because they can shut themselves inside and hide from everyone outside of the box. When I was 32, I shut myself in a closet for seven days and hid from the world. Many people would say my closet was just a larger box. Most depressives are able to relate to the comfort experienced by disappearing to a secluded place. Isolation becomes a familiar friend and invisibility represents safety to someone with depression. For some depressives, suicide becomes the ultimate disappearing act.

Suicide attempts are either impulsive or premeditated. Impulsive suicides still require prior contemplation; however, the opportunity is unexpected and often follows some catastrophic event in the individual's life. Impulse suicides typically occur with less than five minutes of contemplation and alcohol or drugs often play a part. My second suicide attempt by electrocution was of the impulsive type, and I was under the influence of alcohol at the time.

Premeditated suicide involves planning. Taking your own life is a big deal and many people plan it out days, and even weeks, in advance. Like a magician's disappearing act, suicidal individuals plan the big event down to the smallest detail, sometimes even going so far as to practice. Planning usually involves choosing the place, the time, and the method. It may also include ensuring everything needed is available (gun, rope, pills), and it may involve making sure the person will be alone and have sufficient time to complete the act. Finally, planning may go as far as putting affairs in order, saying goodbye to loved ones, and even giving away favorite possessions. My first suicide attempt by driving off a cliff was premeditated; I planned it almost a week in advance and spent a good portion of the time telling others goodbye.

One of the questions counselors and hotlines are trained to ask is, "Do you have a plan?" A friend of mine tells the story of when she called the suicide hotline during a particularly bad episode and the counselor asked her the question, "Do you have a plan?" She laughs when she recounts how she responded by shouting into the phone, "Of course I have a plan, I wouldn't be calling you if I didn't." The story illustrates that when you are on the receiving end, 'the question' can seem really stupid at the time. That doesn't make the question any less important.

The reason it's so important to know if the person has a plan is it attests to how far down the dark hole he or she has gone. Having a plan means the individual has crossed a dangerous line. It means he or she has gone from the idea to the action stage. For many people, when they reach the point where they have a plan, they are often no longer able to ask for help. Obviously, it's a good idea to seek help before getting that far. Having a plan means the seduction is almost complete.

Seduced by the Solution

The dictionary defines the word seduce to mean, "to lead astray, usually by persuasion or false promises." I don't think I've ever heard a better description of suicidal thoughts. Suicidal thoughts have the power to seduce, to captivate, and to mesmerize. They can give a depressive hope where before there was none. Suicidal thoughts promise an end to pain and an end to suffering. Suicidal thoughts are the Beast's favorite weapon.

Like the Sirens of Greek mythology whose voices lured sailors to their death, suicidal thoughts blind the depressive to alternative solutions. Suicide appears as a light at the end of the tunnel, an open door when all others have been slammed shut. Is it any wonder that so many depressives throughout history have listened to the Sirens' call?

Every time I hear someone say, "Suicide is a permanent solution to a temporary problem," I want to slap the person. Although these people mean well, they don't seem to realize it's the "permanency" that makes suicide so seductive. Not having to face life's problems anymore can appear very attractive, and solving every problem with a single act has its appeal. Suicide is easy; it's life that's hard.

When someone is able to resist suicidal thoughts and say, "I am not going to give in to the seduction today," I congratulate that person. It takes tremendous courage and strength to consider suicide and not act. It's akin to someone offering you the answers to a test, and turning them down stating, "Good or bad, I'm going to earn my own grade." When someone resists taking his or her own life, that person is saying, "I'm not through fighting, I haven't stopped trying yet." That individual should be commended for his or her courage.

Why is it then that so many normal people want to chastise and scold someone who admits they are suicidal? What the suicidal individual needs to hear is, "That's awesome you are resisting the thoughts," or "How can I help?" What the depressive often hears instead is, "How can you be so selfish?" or "Promise me you won't do anything stupid?" It's important to remember when non-depressives make one of these latter comments, that they don't understand the seduction; they've never heard the voice of the Beast.

When suicidal thoughts begin to seduce us, we must remember that the Beast's goal is to lead us astray. We already know that depression clouds our thinking and impairs our ability to make good decisions. Why would we assume that suicidal thoughts are any different? The very nature of seduction is to convince us to do something that what we wouldn't normally do if allowed to think on our own.

The Courage to Say No

At age 17, I tried to end my life by driving off a cliff; at the last moment I slammed on the brakes before driving off the edge. Afterward, I felt ashamed for what I saw as my own weakness, my inability to follow through. I couldn't even succeed at killing myself; it felt like just another failure in a long line of failures. Even then, the Beast sought to steal my successes. What I should have felt was elated, relieved, and full of pride for having one sensible thought make its way through my fog. Unfortunately, I didn't know at the time that saying "no" takes courage.

When every thought, every breath, and every heartbeat screams at you to kill yourself, it can be difficult to hear anything else. Add to that the belief that confiding in someone will draw criticism and judgment, and resisting suicidal thoughts can seem like a battle that is lost from the start. These are the very reasons that resisting the Beast demonstrates so much courage. I admit it's frustrating when normal people neither recognize, nor credit the effort a depressive puts forth in resisting his or her suicidal thoughts. But then again, normal people aren't the ones fighting the war against depression. They don't know how strong the Beast can be.

In a perfect world, instead of feeling ashamed, individuals who survive their suicidal thoughts would be given medals. Resisting the seduction is a big deal; it says, "I haven't quit fighting." I wish more people knew how commendable that is. I sometimes think suicide attempt survivors should wear t-shirts with the simple phrase, "I am a Survivor" printed across the front.

Unfortunately, it's not a perfect world; if it were, the Beast would not even exist. When someone is dying from cancer, he or she is admired for the efforts they put forth in resisting the disease, and the individual is encouraged to keep fighting. Sadly, when someone is suicidal, he or she is often treated as a criminal and locked up or placed on "suicide watch." In an imperfect world, people fear what they don't understand.

Saying no to suicide in the face of all this can seem daunting. Anyone who believes resisting suicidal thoughts is easy has never stood in a depressive's shoes. However, living with Major Depression also turns us into fighters. Threatened by the Beast, year after year, we learn to pick our battles. Resisting suicidal thoughts is a battle worth fighting. The greatest weapon we have in our arsenal is time. Given enough time, we can outwait our destructive thoughts. The Beast will go back in his cave.

Recognizing when the dark clouds are beginning to roll in is a major part of the resistance. Taking proactive steps to survive the storm is the best way to ride it out; once the seduction sets in it is much harder to see clearly. Admitting that suicidal thoughts could become a problem, especially if you've never had them before, can be difficult.

Social stigmas and religious beliefs have beat into our heads the idea that suicide is evil; that those who take their own lives are forever damned. For someone to self-acknowledge that he or she is capable of suicide takes a great deal of courage. It helps to remember that every person throughout history who has taken his or her own life, at one point, believed he or she was incapable of such an act.

Living to Fight Another Day

The first storm is the most difficult; we're not yet aware of how black it can get. No one realizes he or she is capable of suicidal thoughts until the first time the thoughts appear. This may sound obvious; however, the statement makes the point that preparing a defense is difficult when you don't know the war is coming. Once the suicidal thoughts have come and gone (hopefully), having them return is always a possibility. People with past suicide attempts represent the highest risk for future attempts; believing otherwise is a dangerous game of self-deception.

Recognizing you are vulnerable to suicidal thoughts is essential to surviving them. If you suffer from Major Depression, you ARE vulnerable. No one believes it can happen to them until it happens. An individual with Major Depression denying he or she is capable of suicide, is akin to someone running into traffic and believing he or she can't possibly be hit.

Not every depressive will attempt suicide; 15% of all individuals diagnosed with Major Depressive Disorder will attempt suicide at least once in their life.[20] It is probable that number is higher when considering undiagnosed depressives. In high school surveys, teens reported that 1 in 5 have thought about suicide, 1 in 6 have made a plan, and 1 in 12 have attempted suicide in the previous year.[20] Never doubt for a moment that suicide is a weapon in the Beast's arsenal.

There is no shame in admitting you've had suicidal thoughts. They aren't going to lock you up and put you in a strait jacket simply because you have the courage to confide your secret. I won't promise you others will understand, quite the contrary, many people will be immediately alarmed. They may show you a deer-in-the-headlights look as their minds race, wondering what to do next. However, there are many individuals who do understand and can help.

I have found a very helpful statement to be, "I'm having thoughts of killing myself; I believe I need to see a professional counselor." This allows you to voice the thoughts (while you still can), and provides the person you tell. direction on what to do next (help you find a counselor). Keeping quiet about your suicidal thoughts is the worst thing you can do, because it allows the seduction to continue. The early you can halt the thoughts, the better chance you have of not following through with them.

The best tool against suicidal thoughts, is the knowledge that they will pass if we give them enough time. Time is in our favor. Most people who experience suicidal thoughts, only have them for a few minutes, hours, or at most, a couple of weeks at a time. If we can hold on, eventually the thoughts will retreat into the darkness. That doesn't mean our suicidal thoughts won't return; this is a war that is won one battle at a time. However, it does mean we recognize that each new assault will eventually pass.

Whenever I am asked by someone what to do when they meet someone who is suicidal, my response is always, "get them to tomorrow." If the thoughts are still there tomorrow, then set your sights on the next day. The adage, "One day at a time," is often the lifeline a suicidal individual needs to survive his or her thoughts. Eventually the person will wake up one day and no longer feel the compulsion to end his or her life.

Taboo Topic

Suicide is an extremely uncomfortable topic for most people. If you want to see a room go quiet, start a discussion on suicide, and most people will immediately stop talking and begin to squirm. The negative stigma surrounding suicide produces a fear in most people that makes them very uneasy. Not talking, or changing the subject, are ways in which individuals seek to regain their comfort levels. Talking about the taboo is never easy.

The irony is that someone with suicidal thoughts needs to talk about it, and the negative stigma associated with suicide makes it difficult to find anyone willing to listen. A good rule to remember is, when confiding in someone about your suicidal thoughts, keep in mind it is almost as difficult for the other person as it is for you.

Often suicidal people "drop hints" about their intent before they attempt suicide. The problem with "hints" is that non-depressives are desperate to believe the hints mean something else. The subject of suicide is so uncomfortable to non-depressives that any other meaning is preferable. Hints are a poor form of communication; directness is always more desirable.

Confiding Our Dark Secrets

Confiding our deepest, darkest secrets goes against everything we have taught ourselves. To begin with, it doesn't feel safe. When someone with Major Depression spends a lifetime perfecting his or her "happy mask," taking off the mask is a very frightening prospect. How will people react? Will they believe me? Often the reaction I receive when I disclose my depression is, "But you always seem so happy." Confiding our secret means we must let someone see beneath our mask.

Another barrier to confiding in someone, is the Beast telling us to remain quiet. Our depression tells us to hide our secret at all cost; to present the happy mask we have perfected so well. It is important to realize that this is part of the seduction. Accepting that depression skews our thinking, hopefully suggests to us that ideas of hiding our suicidal thoughts cannot be trusted.

Confiding our depression and suicidal thoughts to others is an important tool for coping with Major Depressive Disorder. Telling someone about our suicidal thoughts serves three major purposes: 1) It lets someone else know there is a problem and we need help; 2) It initiates the process of our receiving counseling; and 3) It is harder to go through with our suicidal thoughts once we have disclosed them to someone else.

Our biggest challenge, when it comes to suicidal thoughts, is the seduction the Beast tries to work on us; our best weapon is confiding in others. Confiding in others buys us time, and time is our best ally. Given enough time, the moment will pass, and we will hopefully live to fight another day.

The Semicolon Project

Over the last several years there has been a movement among depressives and suicide attempt survivors, to identify ourselves to each other. The semicolon project was started in 2013 and is about bringing depression, suicide, and addiction out in the open.[21] A semicolon is the punctuation mark used for continuing the sentence instead of ending it. The semicolon movement represents the same thing with our lives; we had the chance to end it and we chose not to.

The movement started with individuals drawing semicolons on their wrists with markers, and has evolved into a worldwide movement of identification through semicolon tattoos. For far too long, depressives have felt the need to hide their disorder; the semicolon tattoo tells others that we are not ashamed of who we are, and that we are proud we are still alive. The next time you see someone with a semicolon tattoo, congratulate him or her for having the courage to continue the sentence.

There is a picture of my semicolon tattoo on the back cover of this book. The next time you see someone with this tattoo, please congratulate them on not giving in to their suicidal thoughts. It took a lot of courage for the individual to get the tattoo, let him or her know that you support their fight. It's time we take away the shame of the disease and treat it like any other chronic illness, something to be acknowledges and treated. It's time to expose the Beast for what he is.

Chapter 7
Sheep's Clothing
Alcohol Lies

Alcohol is the great deceiver. It promises popularity, pleasure, escape, and freedom from pain ... and in the end, it delivers none of these. In just the United States alone, over 18 million people, 1 out of every 12, suffers from alcohol abuse or dependence.[22] That is a lot of deceived people. An old saying goes, "A man takes a drink, the drink takes a drink, the drink takes the man." Alcohol promises you the world and delivers you hell on earth.

When I was a teenager I learned that alcohol gave me courage. I didn't know how to talk to people, I felt I was different from those around me, and I believed that I was somehow inferior to everyone. I would later learn that I felt that way because I was a depressive. When I took a drink, it leveled the playing field, or so it seemed at first. When I had a couple of drinks I could socialize with others, I could start and participate in conversations, and I knew I was just as good as anyone else in the room. When I drank, I didn't need my cloak of invisibility.

Alcohol is extremely harmful for depressives. Long-term drinking damages our serotonin producing capabilities[23] (see Chapter 4 for more information on serotonin). Ironically, drinking alcohol increases serotonin activity while we are drinking.[23] Simply stated, this means drinking alcohol increases your depression over time, and drinking alcohol provides you temporary relief from your depression while you are drinking. Talk about a deception, to make ourselves feel better we do the very thing that over time will make us worse.

Using a Depressant to treat Depression

Many depressives drink alcohol to treat their depression; they don't realize that's what they are doing, they just know alcohol makes them feel better. As previously discussed in this chapter, alcohol actually makes depression worse over time. The quest to feel better by drinking alcohol, becomes a vicious cycle of 'feeling better' and 'getting worse;' and the Beast sits back and laughs at our efforts. Unfortunately, this doesn't stop many people from drinking alcohol, either because they don't know any better, or because they just don't care.

One of the dangers of self-medicating by drinking alcohol is that it is a depressant. That doesn't mean alcohol makes you sadder; it means it slows down your bodily functions. Substances that are depressants slow our bodies down, ones that are stimulants speed us up. Drinking alcohol slows down your heart rate, breathing, and your response times.[24] Have you ever wondered why it's so easy to fall asleep after drinking? Now you know.

You may be wondering, 'Why is this bad?' Having an occasional drink, and doing so responsibly, isn't the issue; there are many recreational drinkers who never develop a problem. The problem occurs when someone drinks too often. When depressives discover that alcohol makes them feel better, and that when it wears off they feel worse, the temptation to drink again can feel overwhelming. Because alcohol is a depressant, you essentially start running (living) at less than peak performance. Your thoughts and reaction times become much slower. This is the reason it's illegal to drink and drive; even one drink starts to slow you down and impairs your reaction time.

Hiding from the Beast

Some people drink alcohol to escape from their depression. The Beast is cunning and patient; it's not going anywhere. Whenever you sober up, and you will eventually have to sober up, the Beast will be there waiting for you. Escape may seem to work for a short period of time, unfortunately, your depression will be even stronger once you sober back up. As much as you may want to, you can't hide forever; the Beast knows this.

One of the problems with drugs (alcohol is a drug) is that they eventually wear off. Our body doesn't like foreign substances and will seek to rid itself of anything that doesn't belong in our system, e.g. alcohol, cocaine, etc. To do this our body builds up resistance to fight off the intruder (drugs).[25] The longer you have alcohol or drugs in your system, the more resistance your body produces to fight it. This is called tolerance.

When the alcohol wears off, you still have the resistance in your body working diligently to oppose the effects of the alcohol. When you stop using a drug you experience the exact opposite of the benefits you received while using it; this is called withdrawal. With alcohol, the result is that you become more depressed than you were before you started drinking. You discover the escape was just another lie.

Descent into Purgatory

Nobody becomes an alcoholic after just one drink; it simply doesn't work that way. It happens a little bit at a time ... so subtle that the person doesn't even realize it's happening. That was how it was for me; I never saw it coming. I started drinking because it allowed me to be more sociable. I could meet people, go places, and do things. Because of my depression, I had always felt different than others ... less than. I discovered that I almost felt normal when I drank alcohol. The addiction crept up on me like a morning fog. By the time I woke up it was already there; it had assumed control and blotted out everything.

Not everyone who drinks becomes an alcoholic, however for those who do, it becomes a descent into a living hell. Having Major Depression doesn't mean someone will automatically become an alcoholic, although it does make the individual considerably more at risk. When I was drinking my way toward becoming an alcoholic, I thought I had all the answers. I would later learn that I was just blind to what was happening to me; I couldn't see alcohol taking over my life.

Some people may ask, "How bad could it get?" It can get so bad that you lose yourself. I reached a point where I felt like there was a stranger in my body just going through the motions of living. I sat by helplessly wondering who this person was because he had no resemblance to who I used to be. I reached a point where I existed to drink. I ceased caring about the people and things in my life, they were secondary to my addiction. I lost my goals; I stopped looking to the future. The Beast loves this.

Alcohol Induced Suicide

Every person has a set of brakes in his or her brain. Like the brakes on a car, our mental brakes are there to keep us from getting into accidents. Our brakes keep us from wandering into traffic, sticking our hand in a fire, or punching out the next stranger we meet. Our mental brakes tell us, "You probably shouldn't do that because it's going to have bad consequences." We refer to our brakes as our 'inhibitions' because they inhibit us from doing something. Our inhibitions help keep us alive.

One of the biggest problems with alcohol is that it lowers our inhibitions; it disables our brakes. Essentially, alcohol allows us to follow through with things that in our sober mind we would never do. I used alcohol to help me to talk to people. Some individuals use alcohol to lower their sexual inhibitions. Other people use alcohol to build up their nerve to take risks. Whatever the reason, alcohol reduces inhibitions, which is why it is sometimes referred to as "taking a shot of courage."

When it comes to depressives, alcohol may even help these individuals commit suicide. When someone who is depressed and hopeless uses alcohol, which takes away his or her inhibitions, the result can be very bad. Throw in the fact that chronic alcoholism robs the individual even further of hope, and it is a recipe for suicide. In approximately one-third of all suicide attempts in the US, the person drank excessive amounts of alcohol prior to the attempt.[26] I know that in both of my suicide attempts I did.

What Goes Up, Must Come Down

Wouldn't it be great if you could take one drink and be happy the rest of your life? No more pain, no more depression ... no more Beast. Unfortunately, no such drink (or pill) exists. Your body is designed to remove foreign substances from it; alcohol is one substance in particular that your body does not like. From the moment you take a drink, your body begins working to rid itself of the alcohol. It does this through your liver, your kidneys, and through the enzymes it is producing to counter the effects of the alcohol. This is a greatly simplified version of what happens, but you get the picture. Essentially, your body goes to battle against the invader, alcohol.

The problem is that once you stop drinking, no one tells your body the battle is over; so, it keeps on fighting. This is commonly referred to as withdrawal. Since your body was trying to reverse the effects of the alcohol, it continues to do this even after you've quit drinking. The result is that you will feel the exact opposite of how the alcohol made you feel. Symptoms of alcohol withdrawal include: shakiness, anxiety, dehydration, headaches, confusion and depression.

The irony is that many depressives drink alcohol so they won't feel depressed, yet once the alcohol wears off, they are even more depressed than they were before they started drinking. Alcohol is not a depressive's friend. It tricks us into believing it's the solution, when in fact it's making us worse. Heavy alcohol use prolongs our depression, and severe depression during recovery from alcoholism, is a high-risk factor for alcohol (or drug) relapse.

Statistically, the number of depressives with drinking problems is high. In any given year, up to 20.5% of people with a diagnosable alcohol use disorder, also suffer from Major Depressive Disorder.[27] When the study is widened to include all mood disorders, the number of individuals with both a diagnosable mood disorder and an alcohol problem increases to 40.7%, nearly double the previous statistic.[27] In a similar stud, it was shown that 40% to 60% of alcoholics suffer from Major Depressive Disorder.[28] From these statistics, it is clear a strong relationship exists between depression and alcoholism.

Recovery with a Beast on your Back

I quit drinking when I was 27 after my second suicide attempt; I knew I couldn't continue the way I had been going. Something had to change, or I wasn't going to live to see my 28th birthday. Several people told me, "Once you're sober your life will start getting better." They were partially correct, I stopped being a drunk. What these well-wishers failed to realize or tell me was that the Beast was still there. I was still a depressive.

Quitting drinking is hard. Anyone who told you otherwise most likely never had a drinking problem to begin with. Quitting drinking when you have Major Depressive Disorder, is even harder. It's like trying to rock climb with a 10-lb sack of potatoes dangling from your belt. With each new step, you feel the weight of your depression trying to pull you back down. It was without a doubt the hardest thing I've ever done. It also saved my life.

Depressives who are also alcoholics, rely on alcohol to relieve their pain and depression. The fact that drinking alcohol has stopped working doesn't deter them, they just try drinking more, hoping and praying that they can achieve the same effect. Drinking has become a way of life for these poor souls, it's a means to manage their depression. When many depressives quit drinking, they lose the only tool they have for combating their depression; it's no wonder so many alcoholics with depressive disorders relapse.

It was five years after I quit drinking before the Beast appeared again. I didn't even recognize him at first. I was sober, had a new

100

job, was doing well financially, dating socially ... there was absolutely no reason for me to get depressed. However, depressed I got. In the past I used alcohol to escape my depression, and I was adamant that this would no longer be an option. I didn't know what to do; nothing in my life had prepared me for this. I came face to face with the Beast, without the benefit of alcohol to cover him over. My depression was hideous, horrifying, and cruel; I saw how ugly the Beast could be.

Realizing I couldn't drink the Beast away, I set about trying to understand him better. I began reading everything I could about depression; this started a lifelong journey to understand my disease. I knew my depression was real and I knew it wanted to destroy me. At the peak of that depressive episode the Beast drove me into isolation; eventually I wound up in my walk-in closet for seven days. When I exited my closet a week later, I knew that I had barely survived that episode. I also knew that I would have more like it in the future.

I learned that most of what was written about depression was by individuals who had never felt it. These people were essentially blind and trying to describe what a monster looks like that they had never seen; some weren't even sure they believed in the Beast. I decided that if I were to survive future episodes that it was up to me learn about my disorder.

That was 30 years ago, and I have been learning about Major Depressive Disorder ever since. Many people would say I have become an expert on depression; I do know that I seem to know more about it than many health professionals I meet. I've even met professionals who don't believe depressive disorders and alcoholism have anything to do with each other. I've met mental health experts who believe both alcoholism and depression are simply indicators of a weak personality. I have actually met psychologists who stated they didn't even believe in the Beast. Make no mistake, the Beast is real; ask anyone who has ever met him.

Chapter 8
Weather Blues
The Weather Effect

Sometimes being a depressive, can feel like I am a walking barometer. My depression is a good indicator of seasonal changes; my depression usually gets worse when the weather turns bad. Most depressives notice a change in their depression during specific times of the year. Some years are worse than others, however we know it will happen every year. Personally, my depression seems to sink in the Fall and starts getting better again in the Spring. When the storm clouds roll in, the Beast is riding on top of them.

It would therefore seem logical that depression rates would be lower in the Southern States; ironically this isn't true, the Deep South has some of the highest depression rates in the United States.[29] Depression rates are dependent on far more than simply weather; available mental health services, poverty prevalence, and cultural norms are all contributors to geographic depression statistics. Two States with high depression rates are West Virginia and Mississippi; both are States well known for their rural populations.[29] States with the fewest mental health resources, or which have the least number of mental health professionals per capita, typically possess the highest depression rates.

There is a great deal of evidence that points to a relationship between depression and sunlight.[30] Many things affect the amount of sunlight we get: overcast skies, time of year (longer versus shorter days), latitude (distance from the equator), and the amount of time spent outdoors. It's difficult to study weather's effect on depression because there are so many possible weather conditions; however, few professionals dispute that the relationship between depression and sunlight hours exists. I feel less depression in Arizona, Southern California, or Hawaii than I do anywhere else in the US.

Feeling SAD

When depression is solely related to the change of seasons, it is diagnosed as Seasonal Affective Disorder (SAD). This type of depression is characterized by depressive episodes occurring during a specific season each year; usually Spring or Fall. Remembering that sunlight is a factor, the worst seasons for depression are most likely related to the time of the year in which the area gets the most cloud cover. In other words, if there are more clouds in the Fall, that will be the time when a depressive is most affected by the weather (Oregon). If it's the cloudiest, or rains the most in the Spring time (California), then the depressive will most likely feel the effects of the weather at that time.

Many mental health professionals dispute whether there is even such a thing as seasonal depression, that only occurs during a single season each year. They argue that SAD is merely symptomatic of one of the other depressive disorders. My own belief is that every individual suffering from depression is affected to some degree by seasonal changes; some people are just more sensitive to weather changes than others. One theory is that our depression gets worse during certain times of the year when we receive less Vitamin D, because the sun is out less.

Fake Sunlight

The influence of seasonal changes on Major Depression is so great that an entire industry has been created for producing specialty therapy lamps made for individuals suffering from depression. These lamps are sometimes referred to as SAD lamps; however, they can be beneficial to every depressive. Light therapy lamps are designed to help stimulate the production of vitamin D, which in turn makes serotonin from tryptophan. Light therapy lamps are designed for this purpose; do not use ultraviolet lamps, full-spectrum lights, tanning lamps, or heat lamps for light therapy.

It's recommended that you use a 10,000-lumen light therapy lamp for 30 minutes a day to begin with, and most people report morning exposure works the best.[31] With less bright lamps the time used needs to be extended; for example, a 2,500-lumen lamp would need to be used for two hours a day. In cases where depression is persistent and light therapy doesn't seem to help, many depressives report improved benefit by using 30 minutes' exposure in the morning and another 30 minutes at night, before they go to bed.[31]

A positive response should be noticed between four to 14 days after the light therapy is started.[31] Benefits from the lamps are short-lived, and individuals who discontinue using the lamps, usually return to their previous depression levels within a few days. When the days start turning sunny again, it's usually safe to reduce the time spent using the lamps, or discontinue using them altogether; at least until next the next cloudy season returns.

D Stands for Depression

Another alternative for treating seasonal depression, is through Vitamin D-3 supplements. Vitamin D turns tryptophan into serotonin, much like a plant uses sunlight to convert carbon dioxide into sugar. Without sufficient vitamin D, you may be bursting at the seams with tryptophan, and yet still be deficient in serotonin. Without enough serotonin, you will feel your depression. One of the best sources for Vitamin D is the sun; when sunlight strikes our skin, we produce Vitamin D. When there is not enough direct sunlight, you can still get Vitamin D through certain foods and supplements.

Very few foods are natural sources of Vitamin D. Foods that are good sources include: swordfish, salmon, tuna, mackerel, egg yolks, mushrooms, and beef liver.[32] Because there are so few foods that contain vitamin D, the primary source of dietary vitamin D usually comes from Vitamin D fortified products, such as milk, yogurt, and orange juice.[32] Fortified means vitamin D doesn't occur naturally, however it is added to the product.

Vitamin D_3 or D-3 dietary supplements, are an easy alternative to ensure you are getting enough daily Vitamin D. You can find these inexpensive supplements in vitamin shops, health food stores, and most supermarkets. Vitamin D_3 is measured in IU (International Units) and it is available in strengths ranging from 400 IU up to 5000 IU. For depressives, I would recommend taking the highest IU dose vitamin you can find.

Research has confirmed that at extremely high dosages (Over 40,000 IU per/day), health problems such as renal failure, could occur.[33] The minimum daily high safe level for vitamin D_3 is between 10,000 to 40,000, and most health professionals will suggest your daily allowance not exceed 10,000 IU.[33] Of course, it is always best to check with your own primary care physician.

Staying Out of the Rain

I grew up in Oregon. It rains a lot in Oregon. Oregonians do not know when to come in out of the rain; to an Oregonian the rain is normal. That describes clinical depression very well; to a depressive, depression is normal, we just assume our depression will always be with us. The logical thing to do when you are negatively affected by the rain, is to move somewhere where it doesn't rain as much. Sadly, the Beast tells us that we will be just as depressed wherever we go. The Beast lies about a lot of things.

The Beast wants us to stay put; apathy is one of his favorite tools. When you choose to do nothing, you are in fact giving in to your depression. Although light therapy lamps and taking Vitamin D supplements are helpful, there is no substitute for good old natural sunlight. If sunny climates make you feel better, then go where the sun is. Many depressives choose to live in southern states for this very reason. If moving is not an option, e.g. job, finances, etc., then travel to sunny areas as often as possible. Staying out of the rain is a choice every depressive can make. Staying out of the rain may mean traveling to someplace sunnier where you feel better.

Regardless of where you live, it is possible to take steps to ensure you get enough Vitamin D. Spending time in the sun (when it's out), using a light therapy lamp 30 minutes a day, drinking Vitamin D fortified foods, and taking Vitamin D_3 supplements, are all ways to ensure you are getting sufficient vitamin D. The best defense against our depression is a good offense; be proactive in treating your depression.

Falling Down Again

As discussed in a previous chapter, Major Depression is cyclic. If you have been diagnosed with Major Depression, it is probable you will have future depression episodes. You may be feeling great, standing tall, and riding high, and one day the Beast knocks on your door and shouts, "Surprise, I'm back!" I'm sorry to be the bearer of bad news, however it's all part of being a depressive. The question isn't whether our depression will return, but when ... and how bad.

When your depression returns because of the weather or a change in the seasons, you may experience an overwhelming desire to hide in your home, close all your curtains, and keep it as dark as possible. It's as if we feel that if we can hide from our depression; that it may not be real, or that the Beast won't be able to find us. I used to stuff blankets around the edges of my curtains to prevent any light from spilling in; I didn't just want it dark, I wanted it really dark. I knew at the time that this wasn't normal behavior, however I also knew it made me feel better ... safer.

When the weather causes us to fall down, it's important that we do everything we can to get back up again. Forcing ourselves to go outside is a good start. In the above example, I got over that episode by making myself go out for a 15 minute walk every day. At first, I couldn't bring up the courage to walk in public, so I walked around my backyard. After a few days, I could walk up and down my street. Shortly after that, the blankets came down and the curtains were opened wide. The greatest weapon you have in your arsenal against your depression, is your will to not let the Beast win.

It takes a conscious effort to resist the Beast. When you feel him approaching, you can either lay down and wait, or you can prepare yourself for the storm you know is ahead. Managing your depression is all about being proactive; don't wait until the Beast shows up before you decide to act, by then it's often too late. One of the ways we can be proactive is by preparing for seasonal weather changes ahead of time. You can't stop the rain from coming, but you can take the necessary steps to stay as dry as possible. One of these steps may be moving to a warmer (and sunnier) climate, either for a few weeks or for good.

Southern Climates

I feel better in southern climates. There will be many naysayers to my statements in this chapter; some psychologists say weather has nothing to do with depression, others say it doesn't matter where you live. There are an equal number of mental health professionals who will say the complete opposite. What I know is this, I feel better in warm and sunny climates. No one told me it would be this way, it's just something I have noticed in my life. After my travels, when I finally returned to the overcast skies of Oregon, the good feeling remained for a week or two. Eventually the fog creeps back in, however for a while I almost felt normal. I finally got tired of the rain, and moved to Arizona. I feel normal more often now.

Find out where you feel the best. Be mindful of how the weather affects your mood. When it's a sunny day, stand out in the sun and ask yourself, "Does my depression seem better today?" When you take a vacation to a warmer climate, make note on how it affects your depression. Research supports both sides of the weather debate; I for one, make my own decisions on what makes me feel better. I encourage you to do the same. Only you are the expert on you!

When you discover what type of weather or climate makes you feel the best, try to include as much of that weather or climate in your life as you can. Human nature is to move toward that which brings us pleasure, or removes us from pain; spending time in a sunny climate accomplishes both. Fighting the Beast involves using every resource available. Every effort you make, like counteracting the weather, weakens the Beast that much more. Weaken him enough and your depression becomes manageable. Manage your depression and the pain becomes less.

Preparing for the Next Overcast

The good news about seasonal depression changes, is that since you know when the next season is coming; you can prepare for it ahead of time. If your depression always takes a plunge during Spring or Fall, Arizona is a great place to Snowbird. Planning next year's family vacation? Plan it during your depression down time and take your family to Hawaii.

Explain to your spouse what you want to do and why, chances are he or she will welcome the opportunity to help you avoid (as much as possible) the mood changes during your annual depression season. The mere planning of the next seasonal trip helps us to feel better. The Beast wants us to feel powerless against him. Taking proactive steps to combat our depression proves that we still have some control over our lives.

Even if you don't take Vitamin D_3 supplements the rest of the year, start taking them before your depression season hits, and continue taking them until the season is over. Eat foods rich in Vitamin D (and Tryptophan) during your down-spell. Talk to your spouse and family; explain what will happen and ask for their support and patience during this time of the year for you. Implementing some preparation before the gloomy time of the year comes, you can reduce the effects of depression on your life, once depression season finally arrives.

I often get asked by depressives and their family members, "How do I prepare for the next big episode?" Being a depressive requires a lifestyle change. Just as the Insulin-dependent diabetic must change aspects of his or her life, for the rest of their life, so also does being a depressive require life changes. When appropriate adjustments are made, such as ensuring you get enough Vitamin D, life becomes more manageable. Ignoring the disease only serves to feed the Beast.

Chapter 9
Men and Women
Aren't Created Equal
Physiological Differences

When it comes to depression, men and women are not affected the same. For the most part, women suffer more physically, and men have more difficulty emotionally; don't blame me, I didn't write the rules. The obvious physical difference is that a woman's hormones become hyperactive during pregnancy, menstruation cycle, and menopause. A less obvious difference is that women don't make as much serotonin as men.

Most women with Major Depressive Disorder report that their depression symptoms worsen a few days before their monthly cycle begins.[34] Also, occurring during this time is an increase in cortisol, also known as the stress hormone.[34] These factors lead to additional stress during a time when female hormone levels show increased activity. Men should count their blessings that they don't have to go through this hormone nightmare every month.

Similar changes are noted during menopause when women undergo a shift in hormone activity, albeit a decrease in hormone activity followed by a decrease in depression symptoms.[34] Probably the most talked about depression event for women is giving birth;

113

this type of depression is so common that it even has its own name, 'Post-Partum Depression.'

Statistically, women are twice as likely as men to suffer from Major Depression. This is believed to be in part, because men are less likely to report depression symptoms; probably because of the social stigmas and stereotypes associated with having depression. This alone, does not account for the large variance in depression rates between the sexes. A bigger influence on these statistics is most likely the lower levels of serotonin produced by women as compared to men.

Studies have shown that women produce less serotonin than men, thereby resulting in lower levels of serotonin in their brains.[35] Low serotonin levels is the major contributor to Major Depression; low levels of serotonin account for the discrepancies in depression rates among the sexes. Statistics tell us that women are four times as likely to attempt suicide as men; now you know why.

Social Stigmas

The negative stigma surrounding Depression is so prevalent that it prevents many depressives from seeking help. The Beast convinces us that we will be thought of as strange, or worse, as fakers. Estimates are, that more than half of those afflicted with MDD do not seek help, many because of their personal beliefs about depression.[36] Stigma may result from the depressive's own beliefs that he or she is weak and unable to cope with the depression, or the

114

stigma may be the result of the individual's perception of public sentiment toward depression. Regardless of the source, stigma acts as a barrier to many depressives receiving treatment.

Of these individuals, the number of men resistant seeking help far outnumbers women. Men typically try to hide their depression from those around them; sometimes even from their spouses. Most men are taught as boys that emotions are for girls; that men should be 'manly' and not allow their emotions to show. The male role models in my life never showed emotions; someone close to them could die, and the loss would barely register on their faces. When childhood male role models hide their emotions, how could boys possibly grow up to do anything different. Males learn about wearing masks at a very young age.

Statistically, twice as many men complete suicide as women; however, four times as many women attempt suicide. It's believed that the primary reason for this discrepancy is that the leading suicide method for men is with a gun, whereas for women it is by taking an overdose of pills. Guns are more reliable than pills. It is also probable that many men attempt suicide because they won't seek help for their depression first; hence they suffer in silence until the pain becomes unbearable. I have lost count of the number of suicide victims' friends and family I've heard say, "I had no clue anything was wrong with him" or "He had everything going for him." Most men hide their emotions very well; depressive men are experts at it.

It's also true that many male depressives are misdiagnosed. For some men, their depression shows up in the form of anger and aggression. Low serotonin levels have been proven to be a factor in aggression.[37] Because aggression is more commonly attributed to men, providers are more apt to misdiagnose a man than a woman with anger issues, instead of depression.

Men Aren't Supposed to Cry

Everyone has heard the childhood taunts, "Boys don't cry" and "Crying like a girl." Men are taught at a young age that it's not 'manly' to be depressed, and that it is ok for women to cry, but not for men. Males are taught to stuff their feelings because crying is seen as a weakness. Some boys are even punished for crying by adult role models. A common threat that many young boys have heard is, "I'll give you something to cry about." Is it any wonder that more men don't seek help for their depression?

Women will generally cry more often than men; women have permission to cry. It's not that women's eyes are physically different than men's eyes, because when it comes to tears, both genders are physically pretty much the same. Likewise, crying is an emotional response, and both genders feel emotions. The difference lies in the freedom to cry, when it comes to displaying emotions, women have more freedom than men.

I can cry at the drop of a hat. In fact, I will sometimes cry for no reason at all; the Beast uses this to torment me. Whenever I cry in public I am met with the strangest looks from those around me, both men and women. I always feel like I've broken some basic rule that says, "Men aren't supposed to cry." Who came up with this stupid rule, and where is it written down? I once started crying during a job interview; I didn't get the job. I guess they also believed in that rule.

Crying makes most people feel uncomfortable. It is socially unacceptable to cry in public. When a woman cries, those around her may long to protect her, to comfort her, or to fix whatever it is that is causing her to cry. When a man cries in public, those around him will divert their eyes, look away completely, and sometimes even pretend they didn't see his tears. When a man cries, he is made to feel like he is doing something wrong.

Crying relieves aggression; when someone sheds tears, their aggression lessons.[38] I have a tendency to cry when I become angry; it helps me diffuse my anger. This further explains why depressive men are typically more aggressive than depressive women; many men often have no other outlet for their pain.

Talking About the Unmentionable

Depression negatively affects our sex lives. I wish there was a nicer way to put that, but there it is, don't shoot the messenger. If that's not bad enough, antidepressant medications also negatively affect the sex lives of over 50% of those who take them. Loss of desire, and erectile dysfunction, are two of the more common side effects from antidepressants. Want to improve your sex life? Manage your depression.

Men seem to get the worst of it, however depression affects both male and female sex drives. Men suffering from depression have the added problem, in that they may have difficulty in achieving, or maintaining an erection. Women aren't left out; many depressive women have trouble producing their own lubricant. Having a healthy sex life when you're a depressive can be complicated.

An individual's libido consists of two primary things, the sexual organs functioning properly, and the actual desire to have sex. Although each partner can still pleasure the other even without one or both elements present, for the depressive to enjoy sex, both must be present. There are work arounds if the sex organs don't want to cooperate, however without desire present ... well it's like a car without gas, you can push on the pedal all you want, however, you're not going anywhere.

When you find that you have little to no desire to have sex, talk with your partner about it; your lack of desire is affecting both of you. Sexual problems are embarrassing and sometimes people are afraid to talk about them. Not talking about sexual intimacy problems may leave your partner questioning him or herself, or worse, questioning your relationship. It's always best to discuss sexual intimacy problems openly with your partner.

Some depressives choose to not use anti-depressants because of the sexual side effects. Remember that not all antidepressants are created equal; you may experience sexual side effects with one and not with another. One antidepressant that is not known to have any sexual side effects is Bupropion; talk with your doctor about it. Some depressives take medication holidays, so they can have sex; I don't personally recommend this route. Only you can decide what's right for you.

If the problem is a physical one, such as erectile dysfunction, then there are medications that can help. Viagra is not a dirty word, and it has helped numerous depressives have more fulfilling sex lives. Viagra however works on the physical side and will not work if sexual desire is not present ... the car must have gas in it. Again, speak with your doctor about what is right for you. These types of medications require a prescription. They are commonly prescribed for male depressives experiencing sexual dysfunction; your doctor won't be shocked if you ask for it.

Viagra isn't just for men with erectile dysfunction. Several clinical studies have shown that when women take Viagra they experience reduced sexual side effects from taking antidepressants.[39] Your doctor may not be as familiar with these studies on women, so you may have to enlighten him or her. What's important is that you let both your partner and your doctor know about the problems you are experiencing. Sexual side effects from taking antidepressants do not typically go away on their own.

Women are Social Beings

Introvert vs. Extrovert? Statistically, more women are extroverts than men, so much so, that this has become another stereotype. Women are 'supposed' to be outgoing social butterflies, men are supposed to be quiet and reserved. Where do people come up with these labels? So, what do you do when you are a male extrovert or a female introvert? Answer: you refuse to be stereotyped.

Introversion and Extroversion are personality types. Depression is a biological disorder. It's Apples and oranges. The Beast makes a depressive feel less than ... like we don't belong in the human race; this is not the same thing as introversion. Being an introvert means you are energized by being alone; recharging your batteries if you will. Your personality type is who you are, it doesn't change like your depression. Depression changes with the weather, cycles, medication, etc. An introvert can be a depressive, however the two have nothing to do with each other.

How do you know if you are an introvert or an extrovert? One way is to take a personality test (check the Internet). It's usually not too hard to figure out. Do you need a fair amount of time to yourself (Introvert), or would you prefer to be around other people most of the time (Extrovert)? How can you tell if your depression is actually introversion, or vice versa? Be mindful of how you feel at all times, especially when your depression subsides. If you'd rather not be around people even though you're not depressed, chances are good you're an introvert.

When the Baby Blues Refuse to Leave

Studies have shown that 14% to 19% (1 in 7) of all new mothers, go through post-partum depression.[40] For most women, childbirth is a joyous time that temporarily alleviates any pre-existing depression symptoms. For women suffering from post-partum depression, the symptoms can worsen and interfere with mother/child bonding. Loss of self, feeling unprepared for motherhood, and a previous diagnosis of depression are all major contributors to post-partum depression.

Post-partum depression is dangerous and should always be taken seriously. The Beast seeks to steal your joy. Self-harm ideation is high in post-partum mothers, and suicide is the second leading cause of death for this group of depressives.[40] If you find your baby blues lasting beyond 2-4 weeks, or if you start thinking about ways to harm yourself, it is important to seek professional help right away. Prior to delivery, discuss it with your partner so he or she may be watching for post-partum signs. If they appear, attend counseling with a therapist familiar with post-partum depression.

This Page left Intentionally Blank

Chapter 10
Religion Might Surprise You
Religion Takes a Stand

If you are someone who gets squeamish or is offended any time God's name or the Bible is mentioned, you might want to skip this chapter. Then again, you might learn something so feel free to read on. This chapter is about religion's views on depression and suicide; there is a lot of misinformation circulating around.

To begin with, belief in God and religion are not the same thing. Religion happened when a bunch of people got together and said, "You believe like I do, let's believe together." These people then created rules that you were supposed to follow if you wanted to be part of their religion. Religion could be said to be believing in God with man-made rules.

Most religions condemn suicide. Many religions teach that if you commit suicide you are destined to go to hell. That's one of those man-made rules; God never said that. Some religions teach that depression isn't something real, rather it is demonic possession; these religions should be charged with practicing medicine without a license. A few religions go so far as to teach that if you pray to be healed from your depression and you're not, then your faith wasn't strong enough. These people should walk in a depressive's shoes for one day and then see how much compassion they have for the rest of God's children.

In Christian and Judaic faiths, the Bible and the Tanakh do not specifically condemn suicide, in fact there are numerous suicides in the Bible. These religions nevertheless take a strong position against suicide. These faiths have a moderate suicide rate. Islam goes as far as to say in the Qur'aan that suicide is a sin against Allah and followers believe that suicide is forbidden. Muhammad stated in Sahih Al-Bukhan, "And whosoever commits suicide with a piece of iron, he will be punished with the same piece of iron in the Hell-fire." Muslims have a very low suicide rate.[41]

Hinduism considers suicide to be unacceptable and equates it to the murder of another person; it is self-murder. Nevertheless, Hindus have a high suicide rate.[41] Buddhism teaches non-violence, and the greatest example of violence is murder, both of self and others. For the Buddhist, a negative behavior in this life results in worse circumstances in the next life, therefore suicide is considered pointless. Buddhists have a very low suicide rate.

Approximately 10% of the population in the United States suffers from a diagnosable depression, and 10% of those people will attempt suicide at least once in their life. Approximately 50 million people attend religious services in the United States every week; do the math, about 5 million depressives attend religious services every week, and 500,000 of those will attempt suicide at least once in lives. I pray these depressives will not be condemned by the rest of the people at their religious services; unfortunately, many of them are. Depression isn't selective; it affects people from all ethnic

124

groups, nationalities, ages, and faiths. The Beast doesn't care how you believe.

Forgotten Traditions

In the past, it was commonplace in Christian and Judaic faiths to bury a suicide victim in a separate area of the cemetery, or in a cemetery dedicated to suicide victims. This was done because it was believed that the individual would be denied access to heaven for his or her suicidal act. Likewise, suicide victims were frequently denied any form of religious burial service. It was common for the family to try to hide the reason for the individual's death, so that he or she would not be denied the burial rites thought necessary to gain access to heaven.

Several religions, and most notably Hinduism, taught that death by suicide resulted in the victim becoming a ghost. The living would therefore advocate for the suicide victim's soul, that he or she might be allowed to continue on to the next world. Rituals were often elaborate, with friends and family invited to assist. In modern times, the belief that suicide victims will become ghosts that are destined to walk the earth, has mostly disappeared. However, traditions and superstition continue to keep the rituals alive.

One of the greatest ironies regarding suicide have been the laws making it illegal to commit suicide. Most countries have dropped these laws, although a few still have them to this day. The idea was that by making suicide illegal it would act as a deterrent; all the laws

125

did was deter people from failing. Around the 1960s, individual State governments began to realize that they were criminalizing mental illness by making suicide illegal. Today, no US States have laws making suicide a criminal offense.

Depression Possession

Calling depression, 'demon possession,' has been around as long as people have believed in demons. Through my own faith, I believe that demons do exist, however, I also believe mental illness is sometimes blamed on demons for lack of a better explanation. Depression is something that many normal people don't understand, and unfortunately, some religious people blame demon possession for things they do not understand.

Throughout history, many depressives have been tormented with horrific exorcism rites to 'expel their demons.' Depression and Possession are two different things; the first deals with a biological disease, and the second with evil spiritual beings. Don't let someone convince you that your depression is actually demonic possession (unless it really is). How can you tell the difference? I'm not an expert on demon possession; I have never met someone who was demon possessed. I have met hundreds (maybe thousands?) of individuals suffering from depression. The odds are in your favor it's depression.

Referring to depression as 'The Beast' is a metaphor, it doesn't mean that depression is demonic. Likewise, calling it the "Black Dog" doesn't mean it's canine. Giving our disorder a name, is a way of giving depression a face. It's not real; there is no actual Black Dog or Beast that lurks behind us or in the depths of our minds. Perhaps our tendency to name our depression is where the whole demon thing came from; probably not, the idea of demon possession was most likely just born from ignorance.

Ignorance Begets Fear

People fear what they don't understand; which for some people means they are afraid of a lot of things. Ignorance comes from lack of knowledge; once a person understands something, fear usually disappears. Why don't people learn more about depression? To begin with, many of them don't realize what they don't know. You are most probably reading this book so that you can learn more about depression, there are a lot of people in the world who could benefit from doing the same thing. I encourage you to pass this book on to a friend when you are done reading it.

So why is there so little awareness regarding depression? Part of the reason is that these individuals have had no one to teach them about depression. By its very nature, The Beast tries to remain secretive. Depressives hide from the world and put on masks, so no one will see how depressed they are. We can't expect people to know about depression unless we educate them.

The second reason people are uninformed about depression is because they fear it. If depression is truly an incurable disease (it is), then no one wants to admit that it can affect him or her. If unenlightened individuals can chalk depression up to a weakness, then they can convince themselves that they are too strong for it to ever happen to them. It's kind of like sticking their heads in the sand. Major depression isn't contagious.

What the Bible says About Suicide

This section may not be of interest to some readers; I make no apologies, in my faith we use the Bible and it's what I know. Nowhere in the Bible does it say that suicide is a sin. There are in fact seven biblical figures who took their own lives and the Bible never speaks ill of them for doing so.

One of the more notable figures who committed suicide was Saul who fell on his own sword, so he would not be captured (1 Samual 31:4), and Saul's squire, who after witnessing Saul kill himself, took his own life (Samual 31:5). There was Abimelech, who commanded his armor-bearer to kill him, so he could avoid the shame of being killed by a woman (Judges 9:54-55). Ahithophel, after learning that his counsel was ignored, put his house in order and then hanged himself (2 Samuel 17:23). Samson killed himself by calling on the Lord to give him the strength to bring down the temple on his captors (Judges 16:28-30). When Zimri saw that the city of Tirzah was taken, he burned down the king's house around him (1 Kings 16:18), and finally let's not forget Judas Iscariot, who after betraying Jesus, went and hung himself (Matthew 27:5).

There also was no shortage of individuals who wanted to die; some who even prayed for death. Moses prayed to the Lord to kill him because he was overwhelmed by his burden (Numbers 11:15). Elijah prayed to God to take his life (1 Kings 19:4). Twice Job talks about longing for death (Job 3:21) (Job 7:15), and he even prayed for it (Job 6:8-9). Jonah asked the men on his ship to cast him into the sea (Jonah 1:12) and wished for death (Jonah 4:8). Finally, Paul talks about his longing to die to be with Christ, however decides he is needed more here on earth (Philippians 1:23).

I have no doubt that there are many biblical scholars who will take issue with what I say in this chapter. They are merely voicing their opinions, not the word of God. Personally, I do not believe that God would condemn someone for having a mental illness; in none of the biblical suicides was there condemnation for the suicide victim. In the case of Samson, he sought revenge and there was divine intervention to help him; today he is looked at with admiration for bringing down the temple.

Where did religion get the idea that suicide is an unpardonable sin? St. Augustine taught that suicide violated the 6th commandment, "Thou shalt not kill," and therefore represented a sin at the moment of death.[42] Because there was no opportunity to confess their sin after it was committed, there is no possibility for redemption. If this were true that all sins must be confessed before someone dies, then there are a lot of people who die every day from accidents, illness, etc., without any possibility of redemption; this is something contrary to every religion's belief.

It is more probable that St. Augustine made the declaration about suicide to discourage individuals from killing themselves to become martyrs. A very admirable goal by St. Augustine, however it is hardly biblical. During his time, and even seen today among religious zealots, suicide was seen by some as the only way to gain salvation. Again, this is in no way biblical. Don't confuse the acts of a few religious radicals with the beliefs of the religion.

In the Bible there are numerous instances where Jesus cast out demons from people. During biblical times, there were no names for many mental illnesses. As stated earlier, people often blame demon possession for things they do not understand. It is therefore reasonable to assume that at least some of the individuals who were labeled demon possessed, were in fact suffering from mental illness, and were cured by Christ. It is also true that many of the people thought to be demon possessed today, actually suffer from a mental health disorder.[43]

Has God Forgotten the Depressive?

I can't tell you how many times I've asked myself this question. My depression is a very dark place, and sometimes when I'm in an episode, it feels like God is nowhere to be found. Nothing could be further from the truth. Just because we can't see God doesn't mean he's not there. God didn't create depression, and it saddens him to see us go through an episode. Some depressives may think of a dark episode as hell on earth. If that's what hell feels like (only all the time), then I know I don't want to go there.

Do you want proof that God hasn't forgotten you? The answer is simple, you're still here. Fighting our depression takes strength and stamina. When the world seems bleakest and we wonder what reason there is to go on, we continue to do so because we know that 'eventually' our depression will subside, and we will feel better. Who do you think is giving you that strength to keep going when the Beast is shouting at you to give up? God gives us the strength. In our darkest hour, he is there to light the path.

Does Spirituality Help Depression?

Many therapists refer to themselves as atheists, or proclaim to have no religious or spiritual convictions at all. The irony of this is that 82% of Americans identify themselves as religious, and 56% identify religion as very important to them.[43] Are most therapists part of the remaining 18%? God, I hope (pray) not. I believe these mental health providers are doing their clients a disservice. Counselors are taught that their focus should be on the client, never on themselves. Why is it then that so many of these misguided professionals allow their own religious beliefs (or lack thereof) to influence how they counsel?

Recent studies have connected depression to religious, or spiritual beliefs. It's an inverse or opposite relationship; the more spiritual an individual is, the less depressed he or she tends to be. I think it's ironic that we need studies to tell us this, but there it is, atheists are more likely than religious people to suffer from Major Depression.[44] It's ironic when you consider that one of the nicknames for depression is "The Beast."

Why do religious or spiritual people suffer less from depression than non-spiritual individuals? One theory is that people who have spiritual beliefs, typically enjoy a greater sense of self, and well-being. Essentially, spiritual people as a group, tend to be happier than non-spiritual people. Because depression involves well-being and self-esteem, it makes sense that an individual with a higher sense of well-being and greater self-esteem, would feel his or her depression less. This is not to discount the importance of serotonin and the biological model, it just means that spiritual people cope better with their depression.

Studies have also shown that individuals who regularly attend religious services have higher dopamine levels.[45] Dopamine is the neurotransmitter responsible for pleasure, therefore it makes sense that people who attend church are happier than their counterparts who do not. Need proof? Sit outside a church on Sunday morning and count how many people leaving the services are smiling. Better yet, go inside and become one of them.

Chapter 11
When Someone You Know is Depressed

Depression is a Family Problem

Watching someone drown, and being helpless to do anything about it, is a very traumatic experience; it can haunt you for the rest of your life. You want to throw the drowning person a life preserver, and yet are unable to find anything that will work. When someone you know is depressed or suicidal, it can feel like he or she is drowning. You want to do something, and yet you feel helpless because you can't do anything to help.

Depressives tend to think that their problem is 'their problem.' They don't like sharing how they feel, and they don't like talking about their depression. This can be very frustrating for those around them because in truth, the individual's depression affects everyone who cares about them.

Many people fail to notice the warning signs, they just know the depressive is around less often. The depressive may even drop out of sight altogether, for weeks, or even months at a time. When people do see the individual, he or she is less talkative, may have abandoned personal grooming, and probably will decline invitations to do things or go places together.

When you live with a depressive it is an entirely different story. You are confronted with your loved one's depression every day.

133

The Beast is in your house. When your loved one goes into an episode you will notice he or she goes out less. Your depressive may stay in bed longer, sometimes all day. The individual may shower less often, stop shaving, or cease grooming altogether.

He or she may start keeping all the blinds closed, and the house dark. I once placed blankets around all the windows to prevent any light from spilling in around the edge of the curtains; I couldn't make it dark enough. When you live with a depressive and he or she goes into an episode, it can feel like you are living with a ghost.

Compassion for the Sick

If someone close to you developed cancer would you be critical of him or her? If your spouse was suffering from broken bones as the result of an auto accident would you tell your spouse to 'get over it?' Of course, you wouldn't. Why then are normies so quick to tell depressives to get out of bed and stop making everyone miserable? Give your depressive the same level of compassion you would to anyone with a chronic and debilitating disease.

Depressives don't choose to be depressed; I hate the fact that my depression occupies such a large part of my life. When someone in your life suffers from depression, remember that it's not his or her choice, that person would much prefer being happy. The catch is ... your depressive didn't choose the disorder; the Beast chose him (or her). Having Major Depression is painful; it affects a depressive's life in a multitude of ways. No one wants to feel that much pain and we certainly don't want to share that pain with anyone else.

How do you treat a depressive during an episode? Answer: With compassion. Don't judge us. Don't think we are 'doing it' on purpose or that we are unwilling to help ourselves. Realize that we are sick, and that the depression is our sickness. We aren't asking you to change your life, just to recognize that we aren't in control of how our own life has changed.

Praise vs. Judgment

No one likes to feel judged. Depressives get judged a lot, it's why we try to hide our depression from our family and friends. I wish I had a dollar for every time I've been called Eeyore over the years; people think it's cute, to me it is just making fun of my depression. I don't find my depression funny at all. Every time I hear someone making a joke about depression I cringe. I realize normal people aren't trying to be hurtful … they just don't get it. Normal people have a hard time getting past the false idea that we can control our depression (we can't).

The truth is, if people truly understood what a depressive goes through they would praise us for our strength. Imagine waking up with an intense pain that rocks your world. It's a constant pressure that holds you down and makes every breath, every heart-beat, an act of sheer defiance. Got the picture? Now imagine getting out of bed anyway and starting your day. A depressive in an episode goes through this every time he or she wakes up.

It takes a lot of courage to keep fighting the Beast; you are fighting something you know will never go away. The depressive knows he or she can't win; the best the individual can do is to try to not sink too far; it's like walking across quicksand with a pair of 50-pound weights. This is the reason so many depressives give up and take the suicide path. Staying alive is a lot of work, it is exhausting; succumbing to The Beast sometimes feels easier.

The irony is that when a depressive confides in someone about his or her thoughts of death and suicide, the individual is often criticized as being weak or selfish. When a normie says these things to a depressive, that person doesn't realize how much effort it took the depressive to even confide his or her suicidal thoughts. If you really want to help someone with depression, congratulate him or her for having the strength to keep fighting. When a soldier rushes into battle against overwhelming odds, that person is given a medal. When a depressive faces the Beast every day, he or she is criticized for not being strong enough. We live in a crazy world.

Your Depressive Needs to Trust You

Trust is difficult for someone with Major Depression; we are used to being judged. When depressives disclose their depression to others, we are often met with skepticism and disbelief. Comments such as, "I don't believe in that stuff," or "depression isn't a real problem," are often dumped on us in response. When I receive comments like these, I feel like I'm being called a liar, or that I'm being accused of trying to get away with something. As a depressive I am judged every day.

If you want to help the depressive in your life, you can start by not judging that person. Depressives frequently feel like they have no one they can talk to or share with. Sadly, what depressives really need, is someone with whom they can share how they are feeling. Become the person your depressive can talk to, and you will be able to help him or her through the next episode.

Possibly the worst thing you can do, is assume you know all about our pain. Frankly, it's insulting to us when someone tells us they know how we feel. Normal people will never know how we feel; but that's ok, we don't expect them too. It's enough if you'll just listen to your depressive and accept what he or she tells you. It's ok to ask questions if there is something you don't understand. If we are reluctant to answer, it's because we're afraid of being judged. Gain the trust of your depressive, and we will answer you honestly every time.

A question I frequently get asked by family members is, "How do I know if my loved one is thinking about killing him or herself?" The answer is real easy, ask that person. If your loved one trusts you, then he or she will be honest and tell you. Trust is very important when working with someone with Major Depression. How is that trust developed? By not judging us.

Communication is Key

Most Depressives tend to keep their depression to themselves, because talking about our depression freaks out a lot of people. It's not that we don't want to talk about our depression, it's that we are afraid no one will listen to us, or worse, no one will understand us. Communication is a two-way street, it involves both talking and listening. Listen to us without judging us, and you will hear what we are saying.

When you ask your loved one how he or she is doing, you show you care. If someone is sick don't you ask how that person is feeling? It's no different with someone with depression. The Beast tells us no one cares about us; prove the Beast wrong. Don't be discouraged if your loved one is unable to answer you vocally. Tell your loved one about your day, about what's happening next week, or about the things you will do with him or her once the individual is feeling better. Don't give up on your depressive, we are fighting to not give up on ourselves.

A depressive's main desire is to withdraw and hide; this is also the worst thing for us. Draw your depressive out, take the person for a drive, ask about his or her favorite hobby, music group, movie, etc. Get your depressive through to tomorrow. Major depressive episodes don't last forever, therefore, time is on your side. Help your loved one get through the current episode, until he or she emerges safely on the other side. A major depressive episode is a very dark place; shine as much light on it as you can, both literally and figuratively. Expect your depressive to resist, because the Beast is very powerful. Deep down, we appreciate everything you are doing for us.

There are certain phrases that are offensive to us, please do not ever say these things to a depressive:

- Snap out of it
- Get over it
- Don't you realize what you are doing to me and the family?
- It can't be that bad
- It's going to be alright

Please don't tell us you know how we feel (you don't). Don't tell us it's going to be alright (you don't know that). Above all else, don't ever use the phrase, "Suicide is a permanent solution to a temporary problem." This phrase is insulting to a depressive and was obviously said by a 'normie.' Every time I hear someone say this worn-out platitude, I feel like smacking the person upside the head.

What should someone say to a depressive? Be supportive and understanding. Let us know that we aren't alone, and that you are there for us. The following list represents good things you can say to your depressive:

- I'm here for you
- We'll get through this together
- I'm ready to listen

- I want to understand
- I want to help

Learning to Speak Depressive

I've had numerous family members of depressives tell me, "I don't know how to talk to (the depressive)." If it sometimes seems like depressives have their own language, it's because we do. Fortunately, it's not a complicated language to learn, and you'll pick it up soon if you want to.

Throughout this book, I have referred to people with depression as "depressives." Believe me, I will undoubtedly receive criticisms from professional peers over this label. Mental health professionals are taught to not put labels on a person because the individual is not defined by his or her disorder. I get that. However, it's too much work to call ourselves, 'a person with Major Depressive Disorder.' 'Depressive' is easier to say, and it's how we refer to ourselves. Some people would say the word 'Depressive' is politically incorrect; my response is that I am one and I'm not ashamed of it.

When a depressive talks about 'being in an episode,' we are saying that our depression has gotten worse, and we are having trouble functioning. Most depressives can tell when they are going into an episode. If your loved one tells you that he or she is in an episode, that individual is telling you that his or her world is very dark and does not show any signs of getting better. Episodes can last several weeks to several months.

When we talk negatively about ourselves, e.g. "I'm such a loser," what we really want is for someone to disagree with us. Depressives have very low self-esteem. We see ourselves as worthless, and as having no value. To confirm this belief, we sometimes put ourselves down to see if anyone disagrees with us. If no one disagrees with us, we accept their silence as confirmation that we were right and we really are worthless.

This might sound like a silly game (it is), however what we are saying is, that we need external validation because we are unable to provide any self-validation to ourselves. In other words, we need someone to tell us we are a good person. The deeper we are in an episode, the more external validation we require.

Know When to Call for Help

Never assume that just because your depressive has made it through previous episodes, that he or she will make it through the current one. Many depressives have fought The Beast their entire lives, only to succumb when they got older. The Beast is always there, always waiting to strike. Complacency is one of The Beast's tools, and it is the depressive's enemy.

When it comes to suicidal thoughts, please don't try to help your depressive on your own. If he or she begins making comments such as, "The world would be off without me," or "I wish I would just go to sleep and never wake up," it's time to take your loved one to see a professional. I've heard people say that statements like these are just a cry for attention; those individuals are close, these kinds of statements are a cry for HELP. In depressive speak, these types of statements are a depressive's way of saying, "I'm hurting a lot and I need someone to help me." When the individual stop making the comments, it may mean he or she has decided there is no help coming and is now making a suicide plan. Always listen when someone makes these kind of off-handed remarks, because he or she said them aloud for a reason; the individual is hoping someone will hear.

If your depressive ever says he or she would like to "see a professional," don't dismiss or minimize the request. Instead, make your loved one an appointment to see a professional immediately. It took the person tremendous strength and courage to say it; he or she may not gain that courage again for a long time, if ever.

Even if your loved one doesn't ask for help, watch for changes in the individual's mood. If the person seems reasonably happy, and then has a down-turn where the individual doesn't seem like him or herself, it's OK to suggest that a doctor may be able to help. Offer to the make the appointment, because your depressive may not have the strength to do it on his or her own.

Chapter 12
Life is About Choices
The Depression Continuum

Life isn't black and white, it's an endless number of shades of gray. Although some professionals would have you believe that you either have depression or you don't, it's not quite that simple. There are many theories about depression and one that I happen to like is called the continuum theory. This theory states that we all live on a depression line, each end of the line being the extremes; black and white. The fact is that each of us is at a different place on that line, somewhere between black and white. We are all gray.

Imagine a depression scale of 1 through 10. At the upper end of the scale is the worse depression you can possibly imagine; for many depressives, a 10 represents suicide. At the low end of the scale is 1 and this represents no depression whatsoever. Where would you place yourself on this line? Depends on the day of the week, and maybe even the time of day. Our depression is constantly changing; perhaps because of the weather, life-situations, or the medications that we take, however it never stays at the same place for very long.

Some depressives never get higher than a 7 or an 8 on the scale; others spend most of their time at an 8 or a 9. Major Depression isn't curable; the goal is therefore to spend as little time as possible in the high numbers. What is important to remember is that your depression is on a scale; when you are at a high number you must remember that you won't stay there. Whatever goes up, must come down ... this includes your depression.

Resistance vs. Submission

The fight wears you down. The Beast is relentless, and fighting him day after day, can drain your energy dry. My best advice is never stop fighting; resist your depression with everything you have. Your depression doesn't get to win, don't give in to it. The Beast wants your submission, he wants you to give up, and he will try to convince you that resistance is useless. This is just another one of the lies the Beast tells us.

The dictionary defines submission as: "the action or fact of accepting or yielding to a superior force." Your depression is not a superior force; the Beast is not stronger than you are. Don't believe it? You are still here; you are reading these words. If the Beast were as strong as you believe him to be, your depression would have destroyed you long ago. There were over 43,000 completed suicides last year and you weren't one of them. That shows strength. Choosing to go on when confronted by the Beast shows courage and tenacity. Non-depressives will never understand that ... don't expect them to. What is important is that you get it.

Resistance is often misunderstood. Resistance doesn't mean you have stopped the enemy, it means you have pushed back and slowed him down. The dictionary defines resistance as "refusal to accept something new or different." You don't ever have to lay down and accept your depression. Time is on your side; you can outwait The Beast. Eventually the Beast will retreat ... just like he always has.

How do you resist your depression? By refusing to submit to it. When your depression tells you to hide from everyone and become a hermit in your own house, resist the urge and make yourself leave; even it is just to drive to the store and back. When you resist, you take back some control. When it comes to depression, resistance is a valuable tool.

Holding on Until Tomorrow

Twelve-step programs use the phrase "One day at a time" to help recovering alcoholics and drug addicts get through the day. They have the right idea. When the future seems overwhelming, and when you find yourself wondering where you will get the strength to keep going, focus on today. Tell yourself that you won't give in today; the Beast doesn't get to win today.

Sometimes we have to cut down the time to an hour, or even a minute. Pick an increment of time that is manageable, and make that your goal. When you reach that goal, set a new one; another day, or another hour. Remember that time is your friend. Every minute that passes gets you one minute closer to when the Beast goes back in his cave. Short goals ... baby-steps. How does a hiker complete a long journey? Answer: one step at a time.

Normal people plan their futures; depressives plan their survival. You can beat the Beast; you always have in the past. It's what we do. The enemy is suicide; it is the Beast's favorite tool. Do you know what one of the most important skills taught to suicide hotline workers is? Get the caller through the moment. Set your sights on tomorrow and eventually it will come.

Discovering We Have Choices

I remember the day I discovered I had choices; it was something that had never occurred to me. I always believed I was destined to be depressed, to be an outsider, and to be alone. I never belonged, and I also believed this was beyond my control. I believed that my future was pre-determined and that I was just along for the ride. I know now that I had choices all along, refusing to believe I had choices was also a choice.

I always believed I would commit suicide someday, the only question was when. I felt hopeless and weak against my depression, and I knew I would one day choose to end my life. Make no mistake, depression is real, the Beast is real; however, how we manage our depression is a choice. I believed that picking the time and manner of my death was one of the few choices I had. What I was failed to realize at the time was that 'not committing suicide' is also a choice. I failed to realize I had options.

I have learned in life that I have choices and that one of my choices is to keep living. Another choice I make is to not give in to the Beast. It takes a lot of courage to face a giant, and it is something that should never be looked upon lightly. Contemplating suicide to end the pain, and choosing to keep fighting instead, takes a great deal of courage. Having depression doesn't mean we're weak, it makes us strong. The famous philosopher Friedrich Nietzsche said, "That which does not kill us makes us stronger." Nietzsche was also a depressive.

Taming the Beast

Sometimes I get asked why depressives name their depression, e.g. The Beast, The Black Dog, The Fog. It's because it is easier to fight something when you can visualize it, when it's real. For a long time, my depression didn't have a name or a face, it was just this thing that hid in the background and suckered punched me whenever I wasn't looking. When I learned my depression was real, and that it was an actual disease, I discovered it was something I could fight. With knowledge comes power; my power is my ability to resist the Beast.

Just like taming any other wild beast, you need the proper tools to tame your depression. Doing nothing can have disastrous results; the suicide rate among depressives testifies to this. As mentioned earlier, you have the choice to resist your depression. This doesn't mean you won't feel the presence of the Beast, it simply means you won't give in to him.

Common tools depressives can use to manage their depression include medication, homeopathic remedies, counseling, and having a plan for when the Beast appears. Medication isn't for everyone, and some people are very much against taking meds; I understand this. However, I will tell you that medication can lessen how far you fall in an episode, and shorten how long the episode lasts.

Homeopathic remedies such as Vitamin D-3 are an additional tool in your arsenal. When fighting your depression, use every tool at your disposal. Counseling gives you an outlet for talking about your depression. In a world full of normies, it can be very comforting to to talk about your depression with someone who understands and doesn't judge you.

Having a safety plan is perhaps the most valuable tool you can have. When you're in an episode, it is very hard to think straight; making a plan at that point is nearly impossible. The time to plan is before you start your next episode. Creating a safety plan for a depressive episode before it starts is good insurance to make sure you will get through it. Talking with friends, spouses, etc. about being part of your support, is an important piece of the safety plan. Suggest to your loved ones that if they haven't heard from you in a while that they come look for you. Asking others to hold you accountable is a good way to keep yourself from isolating.

Become involved in an activity that requires you to leave your home regularly. Use a daily pill case so you won't have to remember whether you have taken your medication (or vitamins) each day.

Commit to walking with a neighbor for 15-30 minutes every morning. Plan ways to keep from isolating and hiding. A well-thought out safety plan ensures you are ready for the next time the Beast comes to visit.

The Next Remission Is Just Around the Corner

Just like a morning fog, depression doesn't hang around forever. Eventually it burns off and the sun come out ... the Beast goes away ... for a while. The tricky part is hanging on until this happens. When every day is a struggle, and the air around you is so heavy it weighs you down like a sack of cement, it's hard to think past the moment.

If you are in your first or second depressive episode, it's hard to imagine that your depression will ever end. It will ... the episodes eventually end for each of us. This is where having a support group, or a therapist to talk to can help. When you feel like you're forever trapped in the fog, talking to someone who has major depression, or who has experience with it, can serve as a good reminder that nothing lasts forever.

You may even turn out to be one of the fortunate who only experience a single major depression episode; if so consider yourself blessed. The more episodes you have, the more likely you will continue to have them in the future. The point of this chapter is, plan for the future, so you can plan for your survival.

The darkest part of a major depression episode usually lasts anywhere from two weeks to two months. This doesn't mean you will only feel depressed for this long; it simply means your depression level only remains at a 9 or 10 for this length of time. What this tells you is that the Beast will go away (for a while) if you give him the chance.

When your depression goes away for a while, it's called going into remission. Remission means that the symptoms of an incurable disease have temporarily disappeared. I prefer to call it my up-cycle, because during that time I feel better. I know the down-cycle is coming, but for the time being I'm going to feel good. When you are in deep in an episode, remember that your up-cycle may be just around the next corner.

Practicing Mindfulness

Therapists call it mindfulness, what it essentially means is being aware of where you are on the 1-10 depression scale at any given time. It's about living in the moment and paying attention to how you are doing at that moment. Where is your depression level right now (1-10)? How stressed are you feeling at this moment?

If you are higher than a 5 on the depression scale, what are you doing to bring your number back down? Did you remember to take your medication? When was the last time you did something socially with other people? Being mindful of our depression is quite possibly the best defense we have against it. When the fog starts to roll in, it is time to make sure you know where you are and how you will get out. The best defense is a good offense.

I hope this book has proven helpful to you, or at the very least given you a little hope. Having Major Depression is not a picnic; always remember that every storm passes, and after each storm come clear skies ... at least until the next storm appears. Major Depression is a handicap; however, it doesn't have to rule your life.

This Page left Intentionally Blank

References

1. CDC Features - Preventing Suicide. (2011). Retrieved from http://www.cdc.gov/Features/PreventingSuicide/

2. CDC - Ten Leading Causes of Death. (2010). Retrieved from http://www.cdc.gov/injury/wisqars/LeadingCauses.html

3. DSM-IV-TR.

4. European College of Neuropsychopharmacology (2007, October 17). Depression and Cardiovascular Disease. *Science Daily.*

5. Murray, C. J. (). *Encyclopedia of the Romantic Era, 1760-1850: A-K.*

6. Fromm, E. (). *Man for Himself: an inquiry into the psychology of ethics.*

7. Reynolds, A. J. (). Anglo-Saxon deviant burial customs.

8. Barrett, B. B. (2000). *Churchill: a concise bibliography.* Westport, CT: Greenwood Publishing Group.

9. Hemingway, E., & Baker, C. (1981). *Ernest Hemingway Selected Letters 1917-1961.* New York, NY: Scribner, p. 306.

10. Woolf, V. & Woolf, L. (2003). *Virginia Woolf, A Writer's Diary.* Mariner Books.

11. Qiu, J. (2006). Depression gene in action. *Nature Reviews.Neuroscience, 7*(11), 835.

12. Nurnberger, J. I. Jr., Foroud, T., Flury, L., Meyer, E. T., & Wiegand, R. (2002). Is there a genetic relationship between alcoholism and depression? *Alcohol Research and Health, 26*(3), 233-40.

13. Siegal, A. & Douard, J. (2011). Who's flying the plane: Serotonin levels, aggression and free will. International Journal of Law and Psychiatry Volume 34, Issue 1, January–February 2011, Pages 20–29.

14. Badawy, A. (2013). Tryptophan: The key to boosting brain serotonin synthesis in depressive illness. *Journal of Psychopharmacology* 27(10) 878–893

15. Markus, C. R. (2007). Effects of carbohydrates on brain tryptophan availability and stress performance. *Biological Psychology*, Volume 76, Issues 1–2, September 2007, Pages 83–90

16. Penckofer, S., Kouba, J., Byrn, M., & Estwing Ferrans, C. (2010). Vitamin D and Depression: Where is all the Sunshine? *Issues in Mental Health Nursing, 31*(6), 385-393. doi:10.3109/01612840903437657

17. Julien, R. M., Advokat, C. D., & Comaty, J. E. (2011). A primer of drug action: A comprehensive guide to the actions, uses, and side effects of psychoactive drugs (12th ed.). New York, NY: Worth. ISBN: 9781429233439

18. Ojanen, T., & Perry, D. G. (2007). Relational schemas and the developing self: Perceptions of mother and of self as joint predictors of early adolescents' self-esteem. *Developmental Psychology, 43*(6), 1474-1483. doi:10.1037/0012-1649.43.6.1474

19. Jamison, K. R. (2000). *Night Falls Fast.* Vintage Books.

20. Center for Disease Control. (2015). 2014 Statistics on Suicide Rates.

21. Bleuel, A. (2016). Semicolon Project. Projectsemicolon.org

22. NCADD. (2015). FAQs/Facts. The National Council on Alcoholism and Drug Dependence.

23. Lovinger, D. M. (1997). Serotonin's role in alcohol effects on the brain. *Neurotransmitter Review*, Vol 21, No. 2.

24. Inaba, S. D., & Cohen, W. E. (2007). *Uppers, downers, all arounders*, Sixth Edition. CNS Productions. Medford, OR.

25. Begleiter, H. (Editor), & Kissin, B. (Editor) (1996). *The Pharmacology of Alcohol and Alcohol Dependence (Alcohol and Alcoholism)* 1st Edition.

26. Kaplan, M. S., et al. (2014). Use of alcohol before suicide in the United States. *Annals of Epidemiology*, Volume 24, Issue 8, 588 - 592.e2

27. Pettinati, H. M., & Dundon, W. D. (2011). Comorbid Depression and Alcohol Dependence. *Psychiatric Times*, June 9, 2011.

28. Anthenelli, R.M., & Schuckit, M.A. (1993). Affective and anxiety disorders and alcohol and drug dependence: Diagnosis and treatment. *Journal of Addictive Disorders* 12:73–87, 1993.

29. CDC. (2010). Current Depression Among Adults --- United States, 2006 and 2008. *Weekly* October 1, 2010 / 59(38);1229-1235.

30. Grohol, J. (2008). Weather can change your mood. PsychCentral. November, 2008.

31. Pail, G., Huf, W., Pjrek, E., Winkler, D., Willeit, M., Praschak-rieder, N., & Kasper, S. (2011). Bright-light therapy in the treatment of mood disorders. *Neuropsychobiology, 64*(3), 152-62. doi:http://dx.doi.org/10.1159/000328950

32. National Institutes of Health. (2016). Vitamin D: Fact sheet for professionals.

33. Benemei, S., Gallo, E., Giocaliere, E., Bartolucci, G., Menniti-Ippolito, F., Firenzuoli, F., ... Vannacci, A. (2013). It's time for new rules on vitamin D food supplements. *British Journal of Clinical Pharmacology*, 76(5), 825–826.

34. Baoa, A., Jic, Y., Van Somerend, J.W., Hofmand, M. A., Liub, R., & Zhou, J. (2003). Diurnal rhythms of free estradiol and cortisol during the normal menstrual cycle in women with major depression. *Hormones and Behavior.* Volume 45, Issue 2, February 2004, Pages 93–102

35. Nishizawa, S., Benkelfat, C., Young, S. N., Leyton, M., Mzengeza, S., de Montigny, C., ... Diksic, M. (1997). Differences between males and females in rates of serotonin synthesis in human brain. *Proceedings of the National Academy of Sciences of the United States of America*, 94(10), 5308–5313.

36. Barney, L. J., Griffiths, K. M., Jorm, A. F., & Christensen, H. (2006). Stigma about depression and its impact on help-seeking intentions. Australian & New Zealand Journal Of Psychiatry, 40(1), 51-54. doi:10.1111/j.1440-1614.2006.01741.x

37. Lesch, K. P., & Merschdorf, U. (2000). Impulsivity, aggression, and serotonin: a molecular psychobiological perspective. Behavioral Sciences & The Law, 18(5), 581-604

38. van Hemert, D. A., vad de Vijver, F. J., & Vingerhoets, A. J. (2011). Culture and Crying: Prevalences and Gender Differences. Cross-Cultural Research, November 2011, vol. 45 no. 4 pages 399-431

39. Wang, B. (2009). Sildenafil (Viagra) Treatment of Women with Antidepressant-Associated Sexual Dysfunction. MGH Center for Women's Mental Health on January 6, 2009.

40. Paris, R., Bolton, R. E., & Weinberg, M. K. (2009). Postpartum depression, suicidality, and mother-infant interactions. *Archives of Women's Mental Health, 12*(5), 309-21. doi:http://dx.doi.org/10.1007/s00737-009-0105-2

41. Ineichen, B. (1998). The influence of religion on the suicide rate: Islam and Hinduism compared. *Mental Health, Religion & Culture, 1*(1), 31.

42. Koch, H. J. (2005). Suicides and suicide ideation in the Bible: an empirical survey. Acta Psychiatrica Scandinavica, 112(3), 167-172. doi:10.1111/j.1600-0447.2005.00567.x

43. Gallagher, R. (2016). As a psychiatrist, I diagnose mental illness. Also, I help spot demonic possession. Washington Post, July 1, 2016.

44. Koenig, H. G. (2014). Depression in Chronic Illness: Does Religion Help? *Journal of Christian Nursing.* Issue: Volume 31(1), January/March 2014, p 40–46. DOI: 10.1097/CNJ.0000000000000016 ISSN: 0743-2550

45. Mohandas, E. (2008). Neurobiology of Spirituality. *Mens Sana Monographs, 6*(1), 63–80. http://doi.org/10.4103/0973-1229.33001

This Page left Intentionally Blank

Index

This Page left Intentionally Blank

Resources

National Suicide Prevention Hotline
800-273-8255

Deaf and Hard of Hearing (TTY)
800-799-4889

Websites:

Prevention Lifeline – suicidepreventionlifeline.org
Includes Live Chat

Veterans – mentalhealth.va.gov
Includes Live Chat

Prevention Resource Center – sprc.org

National Institute of Mental Health – nimh.nih.gov

Note from the Author:

If you are thinking about suicide, please talk to someone about it. I've been where you are, and I know it can look really dark and hopeless. You may think no one cares ... you're wrong, there are lots of people who care. I care. You may think there is no other way out ... there are always options.

The problem is that when we get in that dark place, we can't think straight. Suicide can seem like the only answer. It's not. Call someone, talk to someone, call the hotline ... there is help available. The thing is, they can't help unless you let them know there is a problem.

Suicide is not the only answer, nor is it the best one. You will once again laugh, love, and enjoy life. I promise you this will happen, if you reach out for help. But if you take the suicide path, you'll never find out, never get to see it. That would be a travesty.

So, if you are thinking about suicide, please think twice about it. Please reach out to someone, let others help you. Whether you realize it or not, the world is a better place with you in it.

Ron